CHRISTINE

DOING UP
BUTTONS

To Katriona,
With warm wishes.
Thank you for your
time on Friday. In the
process of learning to do
up buttons (put my life
together again) I discovered
a lot about chasing ideas
and capturing & comprehend
-ing ideas.
Chris Durham

PENGUIN BOOKS

PENGUIN BOOKS
Published by the Penguin Group
Penguin Group (Australia)
250 Camberwell Road, Camberwell, Victoria 3124, Australia
(a division of Pearson Australia Group Pty Ltd)

Penguin Books Ltd, Registered Offices: 80 Strand, London, WC2R 0RI, England

First published by Penguin Books Australia Ltd, 1997
This special edition published by Penguin Group (Australia),
a division of Pearson Australia Group Pty Ltd, 2005

10 9 8 7 6 5 4 3 2 1

Copyright © Christine Durham 1997, 2005

All rights reserved. Without limiting the rights under copyright reserved above, no part of this publication may be reproduced, stored in or introduced into a retrieval system, or transmitted, in any form or by any means (electronic, mechanical, photocopying, recording or otherwise), without the prior written permission of both the copyright owner and the above publisher of this book.

Design by Beth McKinlay
Typeset in Bembo by Midland Typesetters,
Maryborough
Printed and bound in Australia by McPherson's Printing Group,
Maryborough, Victoria

National Library of Australia
Cataloguing-in-Publication data

Durham, Christine.
  Doing up buttons : a deeply personal yet practical account of understanding head injury

  ISBN 0 14 026206 7.

  1. Durham, Christine. 2. Head – Wounds and injuries –
  Popular works. 3. Brain – Wounds and injuries – Popular
  works. I. Title.

617.51044

Passing By

Peter, thank you for giving me a second chance with life.
Thank goodness it was you who happened to be passing by.
My St George: you saved me from death, or a fate worse
  than death.
Your cool, clear head was the most valiant of swords.
Now I can watch my kids grow up, I can watch my school
  kids grow,
And my husband and I can grow wise and old together.

To Peter, who helped me live, and to Ted, Helen, Ann, Ken, Rob, Marcus, Deb, Mum and Dad, Greg and Tony for their help, love and encouragement.

This book would not have been possible without a lifetime of inquiry, thinking, problem solving and compassion instilled by my father, the late Marcus Tarrant.

He was a source of inspiration about the power of the mind. 'Chick,' he'd say, 'a problem stated is a problem solved. *Nil desperandum.*'

Thanks, Dad.

Special Edition for the 6th World Congress on Brain Injury, Melbourne, May 2005

Traumatic brain injury is often referred to as the 'hidden epidemic'. People who have suffered from a significant blow to the head can often appear physically normal and in simple social conversations can present quite well. The individuals themselves know that their performance does not match their abilities before their injury. They may suffer combinations of difficulties such as easy fatigue, slowness in absorbing information, difficulties following conversation, and problems with concentration and memory. These difficulties are not always apparent to the observer and therefore the people with brain injury have difficulty legitimising their change in performance at work or in families or socially. Personal accounts of the journey post-injury such as presented by Christine, go a long way towards bridging the gap in understanding and opening dialogue for all participants in the recovery process after traumatic brain injury.

John Olver
Associate Professor, Monash University, and
Director of Rehabilitation, Epworth Hospital and
Caufield General Medical Centre

This special edition is supported by the following organisations:

TAC
Set up to support people injured in road accidents in Victoria, the TAC has seen the debilitating effects of road trauma time and time again. The TAC is proud to have supported publication of this special edition of Doing Up Buttons, confident that Christine's story will bring hope and comfort to the many people in Australia affected by road trauma.

HEADWAY VICTORIA
Headway's vision is that people who acquire a brain injury continue to live as valued members of their community, with access to opportunities and choices that reflect their wishes and aspirations.

In order to achieve this vision, Headway Victoria works alongside people living with acquired brain injury to:
- promote and defend their right to make choices about their lives;
- ensure they have ready access to the information, support and resources they require;
- ensure that the life-changing experience of those with acquired brain injury informs service development, government policy and decision-making;
- fight for the overall provision of equal opportunities;
- raise community awareness.

HEALTHSCOPE COMMUNITY PROGRAMS
Healthscope is a leading and specialist provider of long-term, transitional and respite accommodation and attendant-care

(home-based) services to people with disabilities, in particular those with acquired brain injuries.

Accommodation consists of fourteen community houses accommodating 68 clients, located in Victoria, in areas such as Ivanhoe, Clayton, Oakleigh, Preston, Ringwood, Forest Hills, Bendigo and Shepparton. Attendant-care services are provided across metropolitan Melbourne, Bendigo and Shepparton. Plans are under way to expand both accommodation and attendant-care services to Gippsland and other rural areas.

Brain Foundation Victoria

This organisation provides Commitment Accountability Respect Empowerment Support for individuals and families affected by acquired brain injury, headache and migraine. Contact them on: (03) 9845 2950 or 1800 677 579 (excluding metropolitan areas), or admin@brainfoundation.org.au for information and services

Special thanks to Harry Troedel

Harry, a young man with brain injury, contacted me to obtain another copy of *Doing Up Buttons*. On hearing it was out of print, Harry decided he wanted to get the book republished in time for the World Congress on Brain Injury. That gave us exactly three months and three days to get funding and organise the reprint. Harry made phone calls. Harry sent emails, Harry made connections and Harry did manage to get the funding for this edition. Thanks Harry. Who said pigs can't fly?

Christine Durham, April 2005

Contents

Foreword	ix
Introduction	1
The Day My Life Changed	3
Intensive Care	7
Ward Woes	12
In a Room of My Own	21
Home Among the Gum Trees	27
Spitting Chips	38
Stuck in a Glass Box	42
Out of My Glass Box and into the World	48
Rehab: Trapped in a System that Doesn't Make Sense	50
The More You Do the More You See Your Problems	59
Lorne	64
Uni: Trying to Find 'Me'	68
School: Trying to Find 'Me' (ii)	72
Reality and Unreality Clash	82
End of the Year When My Life Changed	85
In Court	90
As Time Goes By	102
Life Goes On	108
The Good Times Start to Come Again	112
Examining the Heart	114
Facing the Music	122
Mum and Dad	127

The Encouragement Process	*132*
The Year of the Dove	*135*
Postscript: The Wild Goose Chase	*140*

MAKING HEADWAY: SOME THOUGHTS ON CHANGE *149*

HELP SECTION *179*
The Brain and Brain Injury	*181*
You, Your Lawyer and Your Court Case	*196*
Sample Notes for Doctors' Visits	*203*
Glossary of Terms	*217*

P.P.S. THE FOURTEENTH ANNIVERSARY APPROACHES *221*

I'VE DISCOVERED ... *223*

Foreword

I can't begin to understand the courage and endurance Chris Durham has shown in creating this book. She has done something I thought would be impossible to achieve: a lucid, embracing and moving account of the impact of a head injury, recalled out of a mind whose functions had been torn.

This is an amazing story told with a directness that avoids unnecessary embellishment, and a bravery that refuses to shirk the challenge of telling her truths.

One of the most heartfelt days during my own recovery happened when I arrived at Hampton Rehabilitation Hospital and saw those of my co-patients who had suffered a head injury. Their stare looked beyond what they had suffered toward all that was bewildering and lost. *Doing Up Buttons* reaches behind the hollowness of that gaze to help the understanding of all those who face the challenge of living beside, or caring for, a fellow human being who has suffered a brain injury, and all who cherish their humanity.

When I was invited to write this foreword, I wondered how Chris would overcome a dilemma: if a brain was good enough to write a book, how representative of head injury would it be for the many head-injured survivors for whom such a task would be beyond their concentration and mental capacities? All I can say with awe and admiration is that Chris Durham has managed it. This book needed to be written to fill a void: the void confronted by those who endure a brain injury, and the void in understanding of everyone who hasn't.

Doing Up Buttons

The essence of our humanness rests in our brains. It is our remarkable capacities for memory, language, curiosity, flexibility, and, most importantly, our ability to think in the abstract, that separate us from other creatures on the planet. This does not make humans the head prefects of nature, but it gives us unique abilities in creativity, ingenuity, knowledge and individuality.

Imagine that you set out to go to the cinema to see a film. You arrive late because you can't remember the location of the cinema, and because your physical functions for mobility are incapacitated. With difficulty you find your way to your seat. But the light from the screen is too bright and its images blurred or double; the sound system deafening. You settle into your seat painfully, and begin to watch the movie. The dialogue seems to be in a foreign language, the subtitles incomprehensible. And a minute or so after you begin trying to unravel what is going on, the six or eight strangers seated around you begin to fire questions into your ear, seeking details of the plot, the characters, the location, and the action to date.

It was once said, by way of an educational illustration, this is what head injury is like for the sufferer. Partly true, because head injury is not *like* anything.

Chris Durham's book gives us an unflinching portrait of its reality. She has difficulty with chewing and swallowing; altered smell and taste functions; difficulty with speech both in finding and understanding words; double vision and photophobia; hypersensitivity to noise; predisposition to blackouts; intractable pain and unyielding exhaustion; sleeplessness; spatial neglect; spasms, clumsiness and weakness which

Foreword

produce impaired balance, movement and co-ordination; difficulty with attention, concentration, comprehension and sequencing of her thoughts; impaired judgement; afflicted insight; time fracturing; emotional lability; feelings of alteration, alienation, and of being helpless, and useless; and the paradox of needing company, yet yearning for privacy. A six-year marathon still in progress. And yet from within the burden of its recovery this forthright mind has been able to produce an uplifting work.

It took Chris many years to appreciate that recovery from a head injury has more to do with relearning than physical healing, and that the time frame of such a reclamation can be gauged better from how long it took an individual to walk, talk or think efficiently the first time, than from the duration it takes to heal a fracture. She is honest about how her tangled mind and distorted insight refracted her feelings for loved ones – and even her opinions on some therapists. She relates many perceptive moments which will facilitate the recoveries of those who are unfortunate in suffering a head injury, and will reduce the unnecessary frustrations caused by unrealistic expectations and ignorance.

Whimsically Chris admits to the sentiment in a line from *Alice In Wonderland*: 'I'm afraid I can't explain myself because I'm not myself.' She doesn't do herself justice. She has done more than explain herself, she has written a book that will achieve what she set out to do: with a powerful pen she has produced a personal and practical account that will help sufferers, their families, and practitioners toward an understanding of the consequences of head injury.

Head injuries do not happen to individuals, they happen to

whole families. They also make demands on practitioners which at times are both frustrating and rewarding. I am not ashamed to admit that as a practitioner in rehabilitation for many years I was delighted to learn from this book. It is a worthy and wonderful work; a piece of miracle.

Tony Moore
Rehabilitation Specialist and author of
Cry of the Damaged Man and *Echoes of the Early Tides*

Introduction

We were going out for the first time in several months. I'd almost managed to dress myself – I was so proud. What a surprise for the family! I wanted to wear the antique pearl necklace Ted had bought for me in Paris. I'd been wearing it when I had the accident. Ann was about to fasten the clasp when she noticed that there was a drop of dried blood on one of the pearls.

Once we'd cleaned the pearl and she'd fastened it for me, I turned around to be admired. She clucked, 'Come here, Mum, and I'll fix your buttons. You can't go out like that!'

My tiny bubble of self-satisfaction popped. Oh, to be able to do up my own buttons properly! Over the coming months, buttons became a symbol of all sorts of things – small things we take for granted until they disappear – independence, the kindness of my family, being in charge of my life. They stood for putting things together, for size and colour, for skill. My lips and limbs felt as if they were buttoned up. I wanted to unbutton them! But most of all I wanted to button up my life, I wanted to put it together again.

Doing Up Buttons is a story of adventure and love. It's happy and sad. It's full of irony, puzzlement and certainty. It is the story of a journey of self-discovery, and discovery about others, encompassing deepest despair and firm hope.

Since my car accident in 1991 I have been trying to piece together the whole picture of what happened, understand the ramifications and what I should do to recapture myself. People say to be forearmed is forewarned – I was not. There were no warnings of the obstacles and barriers that lay ahead.

I hope that telling my story will help those who are experiencing a life change, particularly those who have had an accident or head injury. I hope it gives family and friends some idea of what it is like for victims to experience their altered states. Professional helpers may get a glimpse of what it feels like to be inside the head and body of an accident victim. Perhaps it will encourage others who find themselves in a similar predicament to discuss their feelings and thoughts with their loved ones.

I urge those who can to record your experiences, on tape or in a journal. This may help you see the whole picture. It's not until we see and understand the whole picture that we can try to put together our new life.

For my last birthday Helen found a great card for me. The picture was of a sweet little pig leaping out over some water. Her words were: 'For the woman who, whilst she can't make pigs fly, can get them leaping pretty far (and there's not much difference!)'. Perhaps 'Pigs can leap!' could be another title for this book!

I hope that *Doing Up Buttons* will, in some small way, help people go forward and put their life together after a life change.

My story has one aim, that is, to encourage. Remember, pigs can leap!

THE DAY MY LIFE CHANGED

Two more sums on the board,
Two sums more, two more seconds
And I'd be OK for sure.

I smiled as I straightened up the postcard on the display board in my classroom. I was feeling on top of the world. The postcard had fitted perfectly into a space among the colourful posters, pictures and clippings I'd put up for our unit on 'Around the world in 60 days'. It seemed unbelievable that I had written it from so far away only three weeks ago.

May 1991
My Dear Amigos, hot greetings from Mexico! How are you all? I hope you had great holidays! Mexico is amazing! My conference was amazing! The reaction of people from all over the world when I read my paper was amazing! The gold and ornate churches are amazing! The ancient ruins are amazing! See – don't forget to use different adjectives! Ted and I are about to rattle through the dry jungle to Uxmal to climb this massive pyramid. Just as well you broke me in at Wilson's Prom. Camp. Fondest love to you all . . .
Chris Durham

Doing Up Buttons

What experiences and adventures my husband Ted and I had the day I wrote that postcard! I fondly thought of the evening of that day, when we had swum in the teardrop-shaped pool as the sun set in a blaze of crimson and a thousand swallows fluttered down to drink the reflected pink water we were bathing in. What a way to celebrate our silver anniversary ... in the land of silver beneath a silver fingernail of moon.

I'd had my paper accepted to be read at the philosophy conference at the university in Mexico City. The atmosphere was exciting – so many people from around the world united in the common belief that the world would be a better place if children were taught to wonder and think. The trip had been a delight, from delivering my paper in the vast hall, to the night when the vice-chancellor gave a party in the courtyard of his home, to the crazy taxi ride across the city, to the deep blue of the sky, the moon and the heart-rending surprise as a Mariachi band burst through the kitchen door. Our Mexican friends had clutched our arms, explaining the words, then the hat would be passed around so we could have another song.

For a decade I had been searching for the magic ingredient that, when added to the school curriculum, could enrich and extend the student's thinking. Like a quest for the Holy Grail my journey of discovery had taken me in many directions. I had studied education and curriculum, and was embarking on my Masters degree to try to find something 'special' that would help my students. I believed that Philosophy might be the golden substance that would enrich our discussions, making them more powerful and empowering. When I learnt that the next International Philosophy for

The Day My Life Changed

Children Conference was to be held in Mexico I was thrilled. Mum and Dad had made travel a vital part of their life and spoke fondly of the elegance, beauty and fascination of Mexico. I submitted a paper and, to my delight, it was accepted.

I glanced round my classroom as I shut the door. What a busy day it had been. It was good to adventure in far-off places, but oh, so good to be safely home. I smiled as I remembered an interview I'd had with the new school principal earlier in the year. We were asked to tell a little about ourselves and I gathered up some things to tell her about my four children. A torn-off strip of white sheet for Helen, my eldest. She'd worn it tied round her arm that summer's day when we'd met for lunch at uni; apparently it was in protest against the Gulf War. Always working for causes, at twenty-four she was completing honours in law at Melbourne University. For twenty-two-year-old Ann I'd taken a beautiful piece of handpainted silk that she had painted. She had just completed a BA in fashion, and was painting, designing, sewing and creating. Ken, who was twenty, was represented by a spoon and a book – what a fantastic cook he was! What a pleasure to have about the house ... so handy and helpful. He was working on his Arts degree and was slightly obsessed with politics. A music note on a slip of paper represented talented, musical, fifteen-year-old Rob. I'd missed his company in the car today – he had to catch the train home from school because I had uni.

I thought of my twenty-eight school kids. It was wonderful to be back at school. I taught Year Six at Ivanhoe Girls' Grammar – a private girls' school – where I'd been for the

Doing Up Buttons

past eleven years. I found teaching fulfilling and exciting. I completed filling the blackboard with fractions for tomorrow's maths lesson. 'We'll finish this unit tomorrow if it kills me!' I thought.

I tossed the bag containing my reports and the papers I'd written for my Masters project on the back seat of the car. It was a calm and pleasant afternoon with the sun breaking through the clouds. I had a busy and interesting evening ahead: first to Melbourne Uni where I had an aesthetics lecture, then I'd grab a bite to eat before my Philosophy for Children committee meeting. As I drove to uni, a sensation of peace and safety washed over me. Although the trains were on strike the traffic was light; there would be time for a coffee in Carlton. The traffic lights ahead turned red. There was no other car on my side of the road. It was eerie, like the calm before the storm. Then I heard and felt a bang.

Blackness. Flashes of bright, piercing, white light, pain, strange sounds of clattering metal, choking, blackness, floating, agony, hell.

Where was I?

What was happening?

A voice floated faintly from far away, 'Is it all right for us to cut off your clothes?' Cold scissors on flesh. Blackness, and yet more blackness.

INTENSIVE CARE

To think I made the news, stopped the traffic, was dramatically rescued, cut out of a car, rode in an ambulance and I didn't know a thing.

The room was dark, but I was lit by a pool of brilliant white light. People were all about me. They seemed to be panicking. I felt calm. Calm and detached. My mind hovered above a tormented body. I could sense that it was me and I could feel the pain and agony. I was floating near the ceiling, looking down at the still body and the people frantically doing things to it. Then I found myself back again on the bed with someone insisting, 'You must make a greater effort to breathe or we'll have to insert a tube into your lungs and you won't like that!'

I don't exactly like *this*! Nothing could be worse than this! I must be dreaming!

This is not happening to ME, a voice inside my head said.

More blackness. Words came from afar out of the darkness: 'You've been clipped. You've had a car accident, you're in Intensive Care in hospital.'

There were painful, yet vague, sensations of being manhandled by different people; each indistinct person had yet another unexpected way to torture me. I was apart yet somehow connected to the weird ceremonies everyone moving about me was involved with. I was central to this hostile act yet unknowing, mute. I was propped up, lain down, my blood taken, tubes were inserted into my body. At one stage, I found myself in the arms of a nurse who was trying to force me to cough and breathe. I had contracted pneumonia. With my deflated lung and the multiple breaks in my ribs I think I was near death.

Sensations of floating through the blackness alternated with sensations of being nailed to my bed, of steel spikes penetrating my body. Each of my keepers fiddled and adjusted the tubes. A tube fell out and blood gushed from the fountain in my wrist. An unseen hand squeezed firmly on the wound to stem the flow. Pain spun up my arm, but I had no words to protest.

Yet another pain surfaced: my tongue. (I'd bitten off a chunk when I had an epileptic fit in the car when I was imprisoned.) But again, I had no words to explain, so I kept poking out my tongue, grunting, and trying to point to it. It seemed ages before someone noticed and painted it with something soothing.

I have had to rely on other people's memories to help me reconstruct the events of the day. Ted, for instance, remembers that Ken and Helen were already with me in the casualty room cubicle along with a cheery male nurse when he arrived at the hospital. According to him:

> Initially the digital displays of the medical instruments connected to Chris didn't appear too menacing and I wondered as to how many hours' waiting we would have before we could take her home.

Intensive Care

'Catch the ambulance drivers and thank them – they were wonderful!' was her initial comment. Too late – they had moved on to another case.

The clothes Chris had been wearing were piled in the corner and I noted that her briefcase carried small segments of shattered glass along the seams. Seems like the car may have a broken window to get fixed.

'I've had a hectic day, the kids were very active and needed lots of attention,' was her comment that roused me from my musing.

'Of course you've had a rough day – a full teaching shift and then a car accident on top of that,' came to me as an obvious comment.

Medical information about Chris's condition remained unclear and unexplained the whole time she was in hospital. Obviously internal damage was involved and the heavy dosage of tube-fed painkiller did not give me the greatest of encouragement.

'Ken and Helen, hop home to make sure Rob is OK when he gets home from school. And by the way, please ring Mum's Head of Junior School with the message that she probably won't be in tomorrow.'

Then began the long and lonely voyage of discovery. Most people will understand that time of stressful waiting as the true reality of a situation unfolds. To those who may judge me as dense of mind, remember that my beautiful golden-skinned blonde wife carried no external damage of note. Isn't the typical car accident victim identified by blood, torn limbs and slashed skin? Besides, there is no greater delusion than the lover willing the loved one

Doing Up Buttons

well. She seemed so coherent and her usual focused self.

The next few hours were spent in the lonely, empty casualty corridor, waiting for Chris in X-ray. A familiar face appeared, Chris's school chaplain. How I now value the expression of solidarity and support that comes from the presence of a friend. The words are often secondary to the comfort of a presence.

Eventually, 'Mr Durham, your wife is to be moved to Intensive Care, please follow me'.

Six days after the accident I had brief flashes of opening my eyes. What crazy world was I in? Spirals of smoke or fog danced around my prone body. Through a hole in the fog I could just see a strange person with two heads. I closed my eyes in disbelief, yet, when I opened them again a similar vision would meet my gaze. Time to retreat into the black world in my head.

I tried to speak to explain this. Thoughts were in my head but they refused to come out of my mouth.

My mind and my body were two completely different entities. My brain felt scrambled, yet somewhere in the depths of my being hovered the notion that my brain was dependent on my body. My body was really important to keep my brain alive. To be locked inside this body that could not communicate was terrifying. From somewhere came the gestures, noises to explain about the two-headed monsters that were inhabiting this horrific world. After some time, a white patch of gauze materialised from the shadows to be fixed across my eye with sticky tape. Blessed relief.

According to Helen, during my first few days in hospital

Intensive Care

members of the family constantly visited, but I was very unresponsive. As I began to realise where I was, I became extremely distressed and overwhelmed by the pain I was experiencing.

I can't remember how the hours passed. About all I can remember was Ted giving me a teaspoonful of jelly and the enormous difficulty I had trying to swallow it. My mouth wouldn't work for talking or eating – was it because of my swollen tongue? Fog continued to dance about me, changing partners with blackness or blinding white light. The music was an unearthly metal clanking, moans and the hiss of machines. Frequently a stranger would emerge from the gloom, crank up my bed until I was in a sitting position, and take photos of me. So many X-rays – I'm amazed I don't glow in the dark!

On the seventh day I was told I was being transferred out of the dark, quiet dungeon of Intensive Care to a general ward. Irrational thoughts like 'Will my family ever find me again?', 'Who is controlling me?', 'Why?', 'Why am I here?', 'Why do I have all this pain?' swirled in my head.

WARD WOES

The pain is as if electric drills are ripping bone and nerves. Can't you turn off the power and silence the drill?

I couldn't see, think or communicate properly. Perhaps someone did try to explain what had happened and was happening to me, but I could not comprehend. All I knew was that I was in horrific pain and this was because I had been in a car accident. I had neither thoughts nor words to wonder how or why. I didn't know who I was, or what day it was.

My bed was moved through a world of endless cream passages, like a giant monster from a movie, bumping and clanging with the attached oxygen bottle, drips, monitors, catheter bag and so on. With each movement it felt as if spikes were being driven into my body The pain of being transferred into a bed in the new ward caused me to nearly black out. I was relieved to be stationary again. Faint optimism surfaced: 'Now it will be a bit better.' But the torturer's rack had followed me. The pain was still there, along with the noise, confusion and chattering people.

My injuries included closed head injury with diplopia and post-traumatic amnesia; multiple fractures of ribs 1 to 10 on my right with right pneumothorax (the abnormal pressure of air between the lung and the wall of the chest that results in a collapsed lung); multiple fractures of ribs 2 to 5 on the left;

Ward Woes

a fractured right clavicle; fracture of the orbit to my left eye; weakness of right arm and shoulder girdle due to a brachial plexus injury, and probable traction on cervical nerve roots; whiplash-type injury to cervical spine; soft tissue injury to thoraco-lumbar discs; and associated ligamentous structures at multiple levels and central vestibular disturbance. In other words, I felt crook!

Ted came to see me in the evening. He tried, yet again, to explain that I had been in a car accident: my car had been hit on the passenger side by a person running a stop sign. I was in a chest ward because of my punctured, deflated lung and the pneumonia that had tried to take me down the tunnel to the 'other place' when I was in Intensive Care.

I lay with the oxygen mask fizzing (what a relief it was when I could have tubes instead of the suffocating mask), a catheter, and a forest of tubes going into my neck to monitor my heart and for pain control. The six-bed ward did not bring peace. The long night hours were filled with the snores of the man in the bed opposite. At visiting time I had heard his wife say that he was the worst snorer in the world – I could certainly believe that! My bed curtains provided me with a some privacy, but with no sound protection.

The pain in my ribs and back took my breath away. It was like lying on a pile of red-hot spikes, and the slightest cough or movement slid another deep spike into my back.

My damaged brain had somehow registered that I was gravely ill. Maybe it is from stories from my childhood, but I knew that when you were very ill you had all your hair cut off to preserve your strength. I managed to get through to Helen that I wanted my hair chopped off. At the time I was unable to even lift my head off the pillow but somehow the visiting hairdresser managed to cut my hair by turning my head on the pillow. I didn't feel any stronger, but I'd be less trouble now.

The ward was a very noisy place. Besides the televisions all competing in volume with each other, there were the chatter of visitors, doctors' rounds and the nurses' monitoring. I asked to have the curtains drawn about my bed, but every second nurse would pull them back and I didn't have the words to request politely that they be kept shut. The light pierced my unpatched eye.

I can't remember eating, and when the drip was removed I don't think I ate for some time. I had difficulty swallowing – I'd choke, I couldn't taste anything, and with both hands feeble, I couldn't feed myself. Neither could I explain what was wrong.

My family visited; Ted on his way to and from work. It was a comfort to have him with me but I felt such a nuisance – he always appeared so hassled, so edgy. I felt guilty for causing him extra worry when he was already going through a stressful time of reorganisation at work.

When the children visited, Helen would massage my clenched left hand or my feet; Ann would softly pat my paralysed right hand; Ken would put his strong hand on my leg; and Rob would look shocked and bewildered. Greg, Helen's boyfriend, sat and read to me short stories by Roald Dahl. Little did I realise that as he approached the end of each tale he would invent a plausible 'tame' ending to the story. Apparently his fear and concern about upsetting me was great, and his endings were amazing.

Ward Woes

The saddest visitors were my dear elderly parents who, at this time, were seventy-five and seventy-eight. They would make the hour-long journey daily, negotiating the traffic and parking and a long walk to the ward to visit me. Looking like two distressed birds, they would search in vain for some slight improvement. Their fear that things were not good, and their love, were palpable. They so desperately needed to cling to something.

Mum would murmur over and over, 'My poor broken doll! My poor broken doll!'

I felt all their fear and despair. I had nothing to offer: no hope, no polite words. I felt a failure. I couldn't fulfil their expectations. They tried so hard to cheer me up but I could not talk when I had no words, nothing to say that would relieve their suffering. I was also very concerned about Dad driving the long distance to the hospital.

One afternoon Mum remarked, 'What a pretty nightie.'

Looking back, she was only trying to find something pleasant to say but inside my head roared the thought, 'I don't care about my damned nightie! I can't see, I hurt, I can't speak properly, I've lost my career, life is awful.'

I'm ashamed to say I told Ted to tell them not to come. I just couldn't cope with their sad, unrealistic belief that things would one day be 'normal' or their need to cling on to some form of hope. I had no patience or energy to pretend I was even a little better. This was perhaps the most selfish thing I'd ever done. I hated myself but I was just starting to understand I needed to put myself and my well-being before everything else in order to survive.

Dear friends, colleagues from school, past pupils and their

mothers popped in for brief visits. It required a superhuman effort to greet them and make appropriate noises to thank them for their gifts and flowers.

I was slowly going mad. The constant noise of televisions and radios, the ever-present nurses, physios, cleaners, visitors and the nurses' insistence on pulling away my curtains of privacy left me at screaming pitch. For hours I would make an 'Arrrr' sound to myself – it made me feel I was doing something, it reminded me that I must be alive.

Ken brought in a Walkman so I could listen to some of my favourite music that he had compiled on tape. Somehow music evoked – and still evokes – how life had been in the past, so that tears would roll down my cheeks and drip off my chin. Ken persisted, and brought in taped stories. He chose Tolkien's *Lord of the Rings*. Words are inadequate to describe the effect this had on me – the sensation of it happening in your head – with goblins and warriors, surreal landscapes and strange happenings all so like the horrific larger-than-life technicolour 3D nightmares and daydreams I was experiencing. I tried to persevere, but it soon became apparent that listening to the radio, music and stories was too disturbing.

I tried reading books and magazines. It was weird trying to do so with the double images, and I had trouble finding the right word and making sense of what I was reading.

The family tried to keep me interested in happenings at home. Rob had a fancy dress dance at school and Ann found time from running the house to make him an Edward Scissorhands outfit after the character in the movie. Rob was brought in to let me see the outfit on his way to the dance. I tried to

Ward Woes

pretend I was interested in Ann's amazing work but I felt isolated, cut off in my own world of pain. Helen skipped lectures to sit with me. She would rub and massage my hand and chat. Ken, who was in the midst of an Arts degree, also missed lectures to sit with me. I needed them, but I couldn't help feeling I was wrecking their lives.

Although I was on oxygen, I had to have my lungs artificially expanded every couple of hours. This meant having tight straps forced over my head to hold on the mask, an excruciatingly painful sensation when my neck felt so weak and sore. Alternate treatments involved me lying on my side to make sure my crushed lung was fully inflated. A worthy and sensible idea, except that when I lay on my side, the large draining tube that was inserted into my lung crunched on the broken bones. I'd made up my mind to jump out the window rather than endure this again. I'd begged the physio to stop. Ted, Helen and my brother Marcus had appealed, but received the same negative response. Our pleas were to no avail: I had to have the treatment.

Throughout the twenty-minute treatment I screamed and sobbed in agony as the machine did its thing with me. The family comforted me, making desperate promises of future pleasures to distract me. When at last I was released from the torture I realised Helen was crying and Ted and Marcus were drenched in perspiration. The next day, I told the physio that I could not endure another treatment on my side. Her reply almost knocked me out of bed. 'Walk around instead, that's okay. Anyway, I've never seen anyone with as many rib breaks as you've got.'

I was determined to walk. My children would accompany

me: Helen would hold the pole holding the drip, Ann the catheter bag, Ken would support me and last, but not least, Rob, like a bridesmaid, would hold the hem of my dressing-gown to stop me tripping over it. What a strange procession we must have made as I hobbled around the corridors with my retinue.

Around this time the medical registrar decided I needed tests to determine what was wrong with my eyes. Only partly clothed in an open hospital gown, with my right arm strapped up to my neck, my bottle of blood, my bottle of wee, the morphine drip and my eyepatch, I was wheeled past fifty waiting outpatients to wait my turn. Fascinated children peered up at me, asking, 'What's wrong with you?'

What could I say? Tears flooded my face from pain, fear and the sensation of being semi-naked in a public place. Miraculously, one of the mothers from school was working at the desk, and she found a blanket to cover my nakedness and moved my wheelchair into a side corridor for the long wait. The last straw came when – eventually – I was tested by two students who spent their time arguing if it was my left or right eye they were examining. A difficult question that could be answered if they only stood beside me in the direction I was facing!

I also needed a brain scan. By now, after so many tests, and being hauled from my bed and put in a wheelchair for the dizzy, nauseous trip somewhere else, I was so terrified that I pleaded with Ted to accompany me down to the X-ray department. I felt excruciatingly guilty about delaying him from going to work, but I knew I just had to have him there. Just to move onto the X-ray table required extra painkilling injections. I was put flat on the metal table in a brusque

Ward Woes

manner. Every bone in my back was shrieking in agony. My paralysed right arm had to be strapped to my body, and in the haste of the action, the broken bones in my clavicle were disconnected.

Having my head inserted into the narrow aperture for the scanning process made my brain just explode; I couldn't believe the fear and panic it caused. At the time it did not occur to me that the fear was due to the claustrophobia I now know I suffer. (My brain must have registered being crushed in the car for forty minutes while the jaws of life cut the metal around me.) I was told not to worry because I had contact at all times with the technicians via a microphone. I endeavoured to remain still as directed over the microphone. I could see them chatting in the booth beyond the glass walls. But it all got too much for me: I sobbed, screamed and pleaded into the microphone for someone to unstrap my shattered arm.

When eventually I was pulled out of the machine, exhausted, limp and almost unconscious, I asked why someone wouldn't help me. 'Oh, we turn off the microphone,' was the reply.

After two weeks of pain, noise, confusion and the bustle of the ward I felt certain I was about to go insane. I begged Ted constantly to try to get me transferred to another hospital where there was a single room, or to the empty single room next door. I had found out about this room when shuffling on a nurse's arm to the bathroom. I wanted that empty room more than anything I'd ever wanted. I would stumble around the corridor and sit in the relative bliss of silence on seats near the lifts. I would hide in the tiny sitting-room and, when I was found, I would beg to sleep the night there. All to no avail.

At last I realised that nobody would get me moved to the single room. Something snapped inside my head! No-one understood my predicament. Even Ted didn't realise I couldn't heal or improve in such a chaotic environment. I cracked. One day when I was in the bathroom I locked myself in and refused to come out until I could have the empty single room next door. Action! Ted was phoned and arrived very quickly.

As he put it, 'Even though in a damaged and desperate state, Chris produced the hat trick. Locking herself in the bathroom and refusing to leave till a solution was found led to the miraculous availability of a single room. Although it was vacated by a patient sent home for the weekend, once installed there was going to be a major altercation to get Chris out. Fortunately this was not needed.'

They say silence is golden. Never was silence more welcome.

In a Room of My Own

I want to be alone!

The nursing staff had refused to move me because I was seriously ill and they didn't wish me to be isolated; they thought it would make me depressed. They thought the other patients would keep me company.

It took the family many trips to move all my flowers and cards from the ward. These things were concrete symbols of good wishes, they were also reminders of who I was.

Settled in my room of silence, I could start to mend.

The pain was still horrific three weeks after the accident. I had been able to get rid of the catheter, oxygen was only used some of the time, painkiller was still administered via my neck, and the physio visited regularly to put 'the pump' on my face to help keep my lungs inflated. In the morning an heroic effort was required to move my stiff body to the shower. To lift my back from the bed using a knotted rope took all my courage and strength. If someone had said, 'Your back has attached itself to the sheet overnight,' I wouldn't have been surprised.

What an achievement when I could shower unaided. I would wobble my way to the bathroom and collapse in the shower cubicle. Sitting on the shower chair I would wrestle with pyjamas when it was time to remove and put them on.

Doing Up Buttons

The sensation of the warm water on my aching body nearly pushed aside, for a fleeting second, the terror, fear and bewilderment.

I could not lift my arms to put on my nightgown. Ann soon solved that problem with a pair of scissors. She split the necklines down to my waist and stitched on fastener ties of tape since my limbs would not obey me, and I couldn't work out how to do up buttons or how to put my legs in the leg holes. I would put on my clothes inside out. The nurses would have to redress me later, but still I tried.

I tried to spend as much time as possible of each day propped in a chair. It was drummed into me that movement was of the greatest importance to stop blood clots from forming and to hold the dreaded pneumonia at bay. Even when in bed I tried to keep my legs moving to supplement the regular injections to stop clotting.

I had little appetite and no sense of smell or taste. When I chewed I would bite my lip or tongue, and the food would dribble out of my mouth, or I would choke and have to painfully cough. Numerous times the tray of food would be placed just out of my reach and would remain there till a kindly hospital cleaner brought it nearer and put the straw in the box of Sustain so that I could have a drink. The kindness, empathy and sympathy of the cleaners were wonderful. I suppose no-one thought of feeding me, and I couldn't think to ask.

Ted was becoming increasingly worried about how little I ate, and one day, he brought in an egg and used the microwave in the nurses' room to cook it. We didn't have a microwave at home, so he cooked the egg for eight minutes then

In a Room of My Own

fed it to me. They say love is blind ... perhaps it's tasteless too, because I managed (just) to get it down to please him.

I felt like such a nuisance to the nurses, who always seemed so hassled. I vividly remember one night being too ashamed or afraid to ring the bell to ask for a bedpan. With enormous pain I managed to pull off my bed-socks, thinking to use them for mopping-up operations, only to realise that I didn't know what to do with the wet socks.

Days dragged on. Pain, clumsiness, bewilderment and difficulties dominated from the moment the bars on my bed were let down. I had to grit my teeth to pull on the knotted rope to get up to a sitting position, then slowly shuffle around to sit in the chair to have the pump and wait for Ted, who would pop in for a few minutes each morning on his way to work. I worried that he was looking so worn out. He looked so busy and hassled that I did not dare ask him to stay. Visits from friends were hard because I found it so difficult to say anything.

Everyday I'd shuffle around the corridors for my constitutional walk and collapse from exhaustion after that. I was bitterly disappointed that I did not appear to be making progress.

Ted would call in again on his way home. As the night closed in I tried to stay awake, to delay the agony of the stiffening-up process of being in bed. Marcus had brought in a six-inch portable television. I would sit propped up on my pillows in the chair, straining to see and hear (after my episode in the ward I was paranoid about disturbing anyone!). I could not understand what was going on, but somehow it was company.

Doing Up Buttons

I'd need assistance to get into bed, and then the bars on the side of the bed would be pulled up. At times the thought of 'What if there is a fire?' made me realise how feeble, dependent and out of control I was. Even with heavy painkillers every few hours, I was wracked with pain. Horrific technicolour nightmares melted out of my pain.

During my fifth week in hospital the remaining tubes in my neck were removed. One evening, a short time after the removal of the tubes and all the sticking plaster that had held them in place, I was trying to tidy my hair before Ted was due to arrive. In the mirror I noticed that the right side of my neck was black. I painfully rubbed the area in vain to try to remove the mark, and asked a nurse to try shifting it with some metho. I was convinced that it was the sticky stuff left behind by all the equipment and tubes, but the stain would not shift. I had no words to ask what it was. I could only wonder in my head, since gestures and pointing appeared to be my major ways of communicating. Weeks later I realised it had been a bruise caused by the seat-belt of the car when I was trapped and choking.

I overheard doctors talking among themselves. They were saying that they would not release me till I was walking well. All I wanted was to get home.

Surely there had been some progress by now? I was off oxygen and the painkilling injections had been superseded by medication. This actually meant that I was in a lot more pain, but it was explained that I might become dependent on the injections. I could hobble about the passageways even if I seemed to miss doorways and walk into the door jambs or

In a Room of My Own

walls by mistake. My balance was terrible: it was as if the floor was a heaving ship in high seas, but I yearned to go home, both for my sake and my family's. I was convinced that if only I could get home I might feel better.

So I entered a new phase where I tried to pretend I was better than I was. I did endless rounds of the corridors; it was so much like walking the decks when I was twelve and my family went to England by ship. Every day I asked the doctor 'When can I go home?', but this request only seemed to instigate a lecture about going on to another hospital, a rehabilitation hospital. I had no clue what that meant. The only people I knew who were rehabilitated were soldiers, and I wasn't one, so I figured the doctor must have been mixed up.

During this time I was experiencing incredible, vivid, technicolour 'dreams' (epilepsy). Reality and unreality were intertwined. I had never experienced anything like it, but I could not tell anyone about it because of my difficulty communicating. I also had the sneaking suspicion that I was mad, and I didn't want other people to know. They wouldn't let me go home if I was mad!

So I fumbled and shuffled and stumbled my way around the corridors, determination on two wobbly legs. I'd walk my way out of the place.

Doctors would promise escape the following day, only to produce another excuse why I could not possibly go home when that day arrived. But eventually, seven weeks after the accident, I was told I could go home. What excitement!

Ken came to take me home. He carefully packed all my things into bags and managed to elegantly balance the wheelchair with me in it, my case, bags of cards and arrangements of flowers on our trip down in the lift and out into the bright winter sunshine.

For a short time Ken left me in the wheelchair, belongings piled nearby, and went to get the car. It was suddenly eerie to be on my own, helpless. But I was alive, the air was sweet, everything sparkled and shone, the mountains were a hazy blue smudge on the horizon. Behind me were the high dark walls of the hospital – so like the tall walls of a castle. I shivered at the thought of the horror and pain contained inside. A woman waiting beside me lit up a cigarette and I nearly screamed at her, 'Put it out! What about your poor precious lungs? You'll end up in there ... and you won't like that.'

But I didn't. I turned away, thankful and astonished at being outside in the fresh crisp air.

Home Among the Gum Trees

I've discovered that animals seem to understand
I've discovered that sunshine on your back is fantastic.

Home. I'd never realised how unique and pleasant our home was. It is perched on the top of a steep slope among the gum trees. The kids had the whole place sparkling and everywhere there were flowers from well-wishers. Daffodils from the bulbs I had planted two days before the accident swayed on their fragile stems in pots on the deck. How wonderful to be home. How incredible to leave home one day and not return for seven weeks.

Our black poodle, Steff, was beside himself with delight to see me. He bounded up to me and Ken had to grab him by the tail to stop him from knocking me over. Within a couple of minutes Steff seemed to sense and understand my pain. From then on he would follow me about calmly. If I sat down he would leap up beside me on my good left side. Most of the breaks to my ribs were on the right, and with my clavicle smashed and my right hand unworkable with fingers that could not move, I felt that my left side was better although my left hand was clenched into a ball and would not obey me, and my left foot dragged when I walked. When I rested in bed the dog would lie on the floor beside me. For the next few months he hardly left my side.

Doing Up Buttons

I staggered around for an inspection. All the time a strange little cloud was following me about, inside and outside. It was good to be home, but in some surreal, strange, way it was and was not familiar.

My smart family had constructed a slope of folded sleeping bags and pillows on my bed so that I could rest while being propped up. Oh, there's nowhere like your own bed, but it was frightening to be in so much pain.

I spent the day eagerly anticipating Ted's return from the office that evening. At the dining-table that first evening home I looked around at members of my two-headed family with a measure of joy and pain. The girls cut up my food and I tried to feed myself with my fingers. I could taste nothing, I knocked over a glass of water, I spilt my food down my front, I choked and coughed. I couldn't follow or understand what was being said. Memories of happy meals, of my insistence on table manners swamped me. I stumbled off to bed. I felt stupid, wicked, guilty, clumsy and ugly.

So me and my pain shadow lived hand in hand. Everywhere I went it came also: in my back and ribs, clavicle and, down my paralysed right arm, frightening pain. I couldn't sit up or move without being dumped by powerful waves of pain.

When I woke up in the morning I was overwhelmed with panic as I tried to work out who I was, where I was, what was wrong with me and what day it was. This sense of bewilderment stayed with me all through the day till I gingerly crawled into bed at night, my senses dulled by painkillers and sleeping pills. The night continued to be a time of terror, when I fought with the wild dragon of pain. Every three

Home Among the Gum Trees

hours Ted would gently and carefully pull me upright (using a sheepskin behind me) so that I could take another painkiller. Many was the time that my arm would go into spasm and I would scream for minutes on end until the pain slowly dissipated, usually after ten minutes.

My movements were very limited, yet I could not be carried due to the intense pain that resulted. Even getting in and out of bed was difficult. If someone tried to pull me up by the arms the pain in my upper torso was excruciating. Eventually Ted developed the technique of using the sheepskin as a lifting band for spreading the pressure and to move me more evenly.

One early morning I was having a great deal of difficulty rousing Ted to move me when he moaned, 'I've just taken a sleeping pill to try to get some sleep.'

That did it. I had spent so many agonised hours at night shaking with pain, hating to wake Ted to sit me up. There had to be another way. By swapping sides of the bed I discovered that I could force myself into a sitting position by pulling on the bottom sheet and pushing with my legs on the wall. What an achievement!

I spent my days wandering about the house, sitting and resting on a bed in the glassed-in room overlooking the valley. Ken cut back the tree-fern fronds so that I had a view of the bridge in the distance, the tree-covered slopes of Eltham and Montsalvat, and the blue Dandenongs beyond. This scene would vary depending on which eye I had patched.

In the hospital the doctors had explained that double vision was frequently the result of a head injury. Sometimes the eyes righted themselves, sometimes they could be operated on if they had stabilised. However, the doctors were fairly certain that even with operations, I would only have a 'keyhole' of normal vision in the centre of my gaze, with double vision above and below. Without the patch, everyone had two heads, three or four eyes. There would be two spoons where there was only one. The doctors suggested I patch one eye to block out the second image. Depending on which eye was patched, the colours were different – the world tilted on different angles and at night the double moon seen through the glass ceiling, or double lights from street lights, would move and wander up and down through the landscape. Months later Ann made me a variety of eyepatches to match my different clothes.

Ted's activities were heavily curtailed through repeated evenings watching videos and reading to me. According to him, 'It was obvious that she didn't follow storylines but this at least kept her in contact with external stimulation and thoughts. Her melancholy was consistent and extensive; something never seen before in such a positive person.'

Helen remembers some 'terrible fights as Mum was very, very angry at not being able to do things for herself, humiliated that her children and husband, whom she believed she should look after, had to look after her. On a number of occasions I would find her sobbing and she would say she couldn't go on and that life in such pain was not worth living.'

Birds constantly visited the feeding tray out in the tree, and at times the bare limbs of the witch elm would be festooned with a dozen currawongs, all singing their mournful song. They moved on to make way for a family of four kookaburras, and later, the amusing antics of two huge baby magpies and their parents. One certainly can't feel lonely with animals about. They gave me some comfort during the long, dull days. I used to lie for hours staring at them, my mind blanked out with pain and drugs.

The kindness of my children was overwhelming. After Ted went to work in the morning Helen and Ann would do their individual tasks for me. It became apparent that the day would not seem so long if I could delay getting up for as long as possible. But with stiffness and pain, staying in bed was difficult. Helen would come downstairs, hop on to the bed and try to distract me with conversation. I was very puzzled that I could not follow or understand what she said and would make what I thought were appropriate noises. It was crazy – I could hear the words but not understand them. I could not remember a second later what she had said, or what topics she had been discussing.

Then Helen would help me to sit up and I would gingerly heave myself out of bed to totter to the shower. My head would spin, I would overbalance and slip, I would go to grab the soap and miss it, I would have the greatest difficulty remembering if my hair was wet because I had washed it or was about to wash it. Was this because of my terrible double vision? I found it strange that I had absolutely no concept of the time the shower had taken. Sometimes I felt as if I had been showering or dressing for a split second, other times as if I had been doing the same action for half a lifetime.

Ann, meanwhile, would have put out a tracksuit, socks and so forth in readiness for the marathon struggle of the day called

Doing Up Buttons

getting dressed. Luckily Rob had a couple of tracksuits I could wear. I was like a child. I wore the clothes that Ann put out, and never thought of asking the girls to buy me some tracksuits of my own. Perhaps we thought I'd be better in a week or so!

With my right arm paralysed and in a sling, even putting on my socks presented excruciating difficulties.

My left hand was not too nifty at doing up buttons, so a tracksuit was better than shirt and jeans. It felt more normal to have the girls do up the zip of the tracksuit for me than do up my buttons.

And so I'd struggle on while the girls prepared breakfast. I ate to try to overcome the floaty, wafty feeling, hoping that my lack of taste, smell and appetite didn't show. In those early days I started to realise that being a convincing actress was going to be of great importance in making those about me feel more comfortable.

I could not express the strange things happening to me and around me; all my energy and resources were taken up just trying to endure the pain and live, move and eat. This was a time just to exist, to try to get my poor ribs to heal. Head injuries and what they entailed would not be looked into for many weeks.

If someone told me to sit down, I wouldn't know what 'sit' meant. I couldn't recognise a glass or a brush unless I saw the object in a certain position. It was so weird. At the time no-one explained to me that my confusion was caused by my head injury. The damage my brain had suffered meant that my short-term memory had gone, so I couldn't remember something told to me five seconds earlier. My long-term

Home Among the Gum Trees

memory was mostly intact, which explained why I remembered my family and parts of my home. However, I'd forgotten where light switches were, and couldn't remember where the tap was in the garden. Because we'd altered the layout of the kitchen ten years previously I seemed to look for drawers, articles and cupboards where they were over a decade ago.

Only a year ago I obtained a 1995 publication put out by Headway Victoria that explains the result of a bad bang on the head. To now learn that difficulty with motor ability and control, balance and coordination, and lack of sensations of touch, pain, temperature, taste and smell, and sensitive hearing are all legitimate problems after head injury has been such a relief. It would have been so good to have known back then about so much that had worried and confused me.

Back then, I felt that if only I tried harder I would be able to see or understand or walk or talk properly. I didn't tell anyone how I felt because my short-term memory loss meant that I didn't remember! I was also loath to complain about what I considered 'small' things.

Lack of distance perception was causing many problems with moving about and smashing into things. Our home is on three levels, with the bedroom on the lowest level. I knew that the ground was at the end of my legs, but when it came to the act of placing my foot on the ground, it seemed to be miles away. These visual and spatial problems made it difficult going downstairs, for example. While I felt a little foolish, holding on to an old broomstick helped me whenever I had to go downstairs.

A head injury can also result in an inability to accurately

interpret visual information. So while I knew the word hairbrush, and I could open the bathroom drawer to find it, I could not recognise it when it was there in front of me. I also had great difficulty reading facial expressions, which compounded my feelings of isolation and guilt.

I was not unreasonable or crazy in the hospital when the noise drove me nuts. With hindsight the scan that showed the fracture to my skull and my double vision should have made it obvious that I needed peace and quiet in order to mend. If I had been sent to a ward for head injuries, perhaps my recovery and rehabilitation would have been different. But we were not to know the extent of my injuries at the time.

I also learnt from the Headway kit that perceptions can frequently mislead a head-injured person and thus they may respond inappropriately. One-sided neglect of my brain explained why I left part of my dinner on the left side of the plate – I didn't know it was there. Months later at rehab, I was taught to move my head to scan my plate or the passageway I was walking down. This prevented more bumps and bruises.

At various times of the day I would hold court amid my bower of flowers in the glassed-in room overlooking the valley. Ann would be busy brewing endless cups of coffee and putting out new cups. My visitors would chat among themselves. I felt strange and detached, as if I was there but not there. I had to act out my part as I could not follow or understand the conversations, so I sort of switched on to automatic pilot. People were so kind – visiting, bringing flowers, food and friendly words – but inside me festered a secret sore. I must be a bad and horrid person because I felt so cold and numb, and not nearly grateful or thankful enough for the kindness heaped on me. I felt so helpless, so alone, so strange.

It was not until 1995 when I saw an advertised lecture on shell-shock that I came to understand about post-traumatic stress disorder. I attended the lecture and learnt that symptoms of this disorder include feeling numb and dazed. You feel depersonalised, as if your brain is outside your body and time seems unreal. You don't know who you are and experience despair, hopelessness, denial and guilt.

Add to those symptoms my own: my body felt as if it was shaking inside. I had difficulty concentrating. My short-term memory was terrible. I felt no-one knew or understood how I felt. I was snappy and aggressive. Little things blew out of all proportion. Day and night, dreams constantly returned me to the horrific scene. I became emotionally numb and tried to avoid thoughts, feelings and activities. I no longer found pleasure in things that previously had given me pleasure. I felt totally cut off from everyone, and didn't see a future worth having. Sometimes a noise or movement would startle me so badly that it would cause a chain reaction and I'd be left shaken and frightened. Many days I spent wrestling with the monster of anger. Not only 'Why me?' but also 'Who did this to me?' and 'Why?'

If only someone had talked to me about post-traumatic stress disorder, and helped me to express what I was experiencing! If it had been explained that such feelings of disorientation and frustration were normal for someone who has been involved in an accident, I might not have experienced so much guilt and stress. Information, psychological support, crisis intervention, emotional first-aid; all of these were needed to assist me to address depression, social agoraphobia, chronic pain and panic,

Doing Up Buttons

not to mention being house-bound, and experiencing marital disharmony and difficulties with employment. It has been suggested that 50 per cent of those who suffer post-traumatic stress remain chronic sufferers after ten years.

Things were hard on the people around me, too. As Helen puts it:

> In the early weeks when she came home from hospital Mum was extremely irrational, frustrated and downright nasty. She annoyed us all as she repeated herself, was over-anxious about our safety and generally found it impossible to relax. Mum was not like this before her accident and while I could try to rationalise the problems she has had to cope with, her behaviour caused friction. At times Mum dwelt upon the man who hit her car. She became upset and often mentioned the man who changed her life. When she was extremely distressed I could find little to comfort her as I found it hard to cope myself. I mourned for the woman my mother was, but I was determined to help her, make the best of what she was left with.

In retrospect I can't fathom out why I did not ask my doctor about my various problems. I can only suppose I couldn't reason sufficiently to put the symptoms all together and realise that there was something really wrong. Perhaps it was because in my mind they all added up to one fact: you have gone mad! In isolation, they seemed like small things, and I hated to whinge. Hope springs eternal, and one always thinks, 'Tomorrow will be different, I won't forget or break things or be dumb – I'll try harder and beat it.'

Home Among the Gum Trees

As dusk approached each evening I would feel fear and terror start to bubble up uncontrollably. My night fear of pain would come again. The minutes would creep by so slowly. I would hear the clatter of the children preparing dinner and silently weep. On a tape I recorded:

I feel so frustrated I could go screaming mad. So many weeks of pain, confusion and dependence. At times I think it would have been simpler on my family (and me) if I'd died, if the blackness had swallowed me and they could be rebuilding and getting on with their lives. At other times I'm just so thankful to have been miraculously spared.

Everyone says how well I'm doing, which means that they don't even have a glimpse of the agony, indignity and horror. How can life ever be sweet again? Did I ever value each second, each blade of grass? Where has my enormous store of hope and *joie de vivre* gone? Life seems so bleak. Will I never have that glorious bubbly feeling that life's wonderful again? That man has destroyed more than my body, he has twisted and crushed my spirit, like my twisted and crushed car. I have lost me.

SPITTING CHIPS

In the wee small hours does Mr X ever think of the woman
  he hit?
Does he resolve to take more care?
Or has the whole episode passed from his mind?

My unknown hero's hand, voice, dragging and rescuing me
From the beckoning black void of death.
And I've never even seen his face.

After I had been home a few weeks, the man who had helped me when I was trapped in the car rang to inquire how I was getting on. He had rung Ted while I was in hospital to check on my progress. Peter had been driving in the other direction. He saw the accident and stopped immediately to see what he could do. He noticed that I was having trouble breathing so he smashed the passenger window and managed to get the seat-belt from around my neck where it was choking me. (This explained the terrible black bruising on my neck.) He asked passers-by to ring the police and ambulance. This quick-thinking and practical man then stayed with me for the forty minutes it took to cut me free of the wreckage. How fortunate I was that he was passing by at that moment!

A thought constantly nagged my mind when I was

Spitting Chips

convalescing: an overwhelming desire to meet my hero, the man behind the voice in the echo in my mind, 'You've been clipped, you'll be okay.' I had to meet him.

And so it was that one of my early trips in a car was to visit this kind man. Peter lived only a few kilometres from the accident site. He was a resourceful and practical person, and endeavoured to shrug off his stopping to help me as nothing. Ted and I were acutely aware that but for Peter I might not be here, or might be in a nursing home. Just knowing what Peter had done for me seemed very important. I must confess that I was a tiny bit disappointed that seeing him brought back no memory of the time he'd stayed with me, although perhaps deep in my subconscious there was something about his voice I found very calming.

It was only after quite some time had passed and we had met on several occasions that Peter could tell me how the whole incident had affected him. Apparently after assisting me he went on home and had a stiff whisky and said to his wife that he didn't think I would make it.

Why didn't the man who had hit me ring to find out if I was dead or alive? I overheard Ted telling someone on the phone that the police had told him that while I was trapped in the car, the man had driven across the road to a panel beater to get a quote to have his car fixed. (Later the police prosecutor spoke of the smash repairer's records supporting this.) I would lie in bed in the small hours crying silently in pain, cursing the man who had so carelessly ruined my life. I would fantasise about arriving at his house and pouring red nail polish, a symbol of my blood, down the windscreen of his precious car. How dare he go about as if nothing had

Doing Up Buttons

happened when he was personally responsible for injuring and crushing another human being?

My bitterness grew, fuelled by people asking, 'What happened to the man who hit you?' Of course, the answer was nothing. He eats and sleeps, and life goes on as usual for him. 'I'll show him,' I thought. It was then that the idea to record my experiences surfaced. Rather than daydream about catching a taxi to his house to disfigure his car, I would record my experiences in a book to let him know what he had done. (To take a taxi to his home at that time would have been impossible anyway.)

Looking back, I can't remember when or how I decided that I couldn't or wouldn't let him destroy my life. I know that one day, many months – perhaps a year after the accident – I told myself that hating him was a luxury I could no longer afford if I was going to conserve my strength to get better. The bad, black days filled with hate were gradually, oh so gradually, overtaken by days when I didn't curse him. After a couple of years things changed so dramatically that I got to the stage of actually worrying about him being forced to go to jail, until a friend pointed out how unlikely this was. These days a week can pass without me thinking or saying his name.

When the family realised Ted and I were visiting Peter, they were keen to meet him too. When I was on my feet a little more Helen, Ann, Rob and Ken cooked a special Sunday lunch, and Mum, Dad and my brother Marcus came to meet Peter, his wife Gaye and their two gorgeous kids. At the time I must have still been pretty wonky, but I can remember a warm glow that was not just from the fire.

Spitting Chips

If I had hand-picked a hero I could not have done better. As well as being practical in helping me at the accident, Peter was the best witness. In a calm, unruffled way, he was able to tell the police exactly what had happened. Peter helped to banish the grey clouds of anger and gloom. He was a symbol of good overcoming bad.

STUCK IN A GLASS BOX

I feel like an alien.
I have to drum up enthusiasm to open cards, read letters, express appreciation.
Am I still a member of the human race?

Life went on. The days and weeks passed slowly, so slowly. I could just hold a pen to sign the thank-you letters the kids prepared. I could shuffle to the letter-box, a very adventurous thing to do. I would try to help the kids by unpacking the top of the dishwasher on to the bench, but I couldn't put the knives and forks in the drawer because I would forget which section they belonged to. I would wander from the sitting-room to the glassed-in room. I would lie on the bed and say 'Arrrr.'

Without a sense of taste or smell I didn't enjoy eating. Every hour or so the kids would bring me a cut orange. They had read in Tony Moore's book *Cry of the Damaged Man* how he had a craving for oranges after his accident. If he ate oranges, I had to eat them too! I still could not see properly or concentrate to read. My ears couldn't stand the noise of a talking book or music. I think my first stirring of a wisp of happiness was warmth: the feeling of holding warm coffee in a fine, old cup in my hand; rays of sunshine on my back; the warmth of the love and care of my family.

Stuck in a Glass Box

Kind folk continued to faithfully visit, bringing good cheer, flowers and food. I was still numb inside. I'd say 'It's fantastic!' 'Marvellous!' 'How interesting!' 'Look forward to it!' 'Fascinating!' 'Fantastic!' 'Wow!' . . . but they didn't mean a thing. It was as if I was locked in an invisible glass box, totally isolated from the rest of the world.

The door-bell continued to ring at dusk for months as florists delivered bouquets from friends and families of girls I had taught up to a decade before. Such kindness.

I was fortunate to have a wonderful GP and physio. They visited me regularly at home for the first few weeks. When I was able to travel the family would take me to appointments and months later, I went by taxi. Hugh, my GP, strengthened both my body and my spirit. Hugh first came to see me one sunny afternoon when I had been home a week. He spoke of car-racing, his passion.

He said, 'It is up to you whether you recapture your life, whether you're out of the race of life or not. The choice is yours, whether you allow this to ruin your life or whether you fight, struggle and work to get back in the car and get back in the race.' He spoke with warm admiration of racing drivers who'd had their bodies smashed, but not their spirits.

Hugh arranged for me to have physiotherapy regularly and Philip, my physio, would visit, sometimes as late as 11 p.m., to help me get my paralysed right arm moving. He explained to Ted how I needed a pulley with a sling attached for my right arm. I could then place my wrist in it and pull on the pulley with my left hand, thus lifting the immobile arm. Ever resourceful, Ted fitted up a pulley arrangement from a beam

Doing Up Buttons

in our bedroom so that I could exercise my motionless arm several times a day.

I did no housework, shopping or cooking. I could not read or follow the correct line on a page, or the plot in a book or newspaper. I could not thread a needle or find the holes to do tapestry, which I used to enjoy so much. I could not see to hold a brush to paint – watercolour painting had been a joy to me. I could not go for walks because of my lack of balance and poor depth perception. I could not tell where the ground was – my feet looked like they were ten feet away. It was weird not knowing where my feet or my mouth were. I had the attention span of a gnat. I did not know what day it was, and even when I was told, I'd forget it a second later.

The family, Ted, and Mum and Dad tried to think up ways to help me overcome my disabilities. They wrote lists for me: 'Today is Monday. At 11 a.m. there is a doctor's appointment. You will need to be ready at 10.30 a.m.'

For many weeks I was incapable of finding the correct clothes to wear, so Helen or Ann would mother me, putting out clothes and helping me dress. After some time I tried to organise myself. They would help by making lists so that I would remember to do things that I used to do automatically: get up, shower, put on socks, undies, check that my clothes were not inside out, start buttoning my shirt from the bottom button and move up the shirt, eat breakfast, take my pills, go and lie in the glass room. Eat lunch at 12.30 ... and so on.

I had panic attacks when the phone rang, so they wrote in clear letters on a piece of paper: 'Pick up the phone, say "Hello, this is Christine, Who's calling please?"' If I needed to ring someone I wrote down the points of the conversation on paper and read out the questions and answers. If I didn't do this I would totally forget why I had contacted the person.

I think one of my biggest disappointments was that I simply couldn't stand music, something I had always had a passion for. Nor could I listen to the radio and television – they really hurt my ears. I could not garden with my lack of coordination and balance, and I could not understand the conversations of my family or friends. With no sense of taste or smell I couldn't even drown my sorrows with food or drink.

For months I cried daily. I wanted to die, to escape from this me that wasn't me. For over a year I couldn't do something as simple as ask for bread in a shop without crying. I wept with despair, frustration, pain, disappointment, jealousy and desire to be normal. I cried because no-one seemed to understand what life was like for me. I was fortunate I didn't get 'face rot' from having a wet face much of the time! Tears were never far from the surface. I cried not at the drop of a hat, but unexpectedly, in the middle of conversations with family, friends and strangers. It was embarrassing and perplexing.

I am immensely lucky to have the kids and Ted around me, encouraging me. Helen had very early on realised that I would have to depend on them for everything:

> As a family it became obvious that Mum's quality of life relied upon us working as a unit and thus each of us did our utmost to support her. I have high respect for my siblings due to the many sacrifices they have made,

Doing Up Buttons

especially my two brothers, who were such assistance to Mum typing on the computer: Ken for being a tireless chauffeur and Rob for the encouragement he so obviously gave her. Ann looked after Mum and ran the household for six months and did not seek employment.

Ken also realised that things had to be changed around to accommodate my needs.

Being strong-willed, Mum was constantly attempting things that were clearly beyond her ability. Often we would find her in the garden or laundry, weeping with pain and frustration, after trying to prune the roses or hang up washing. Our supervisory role was now greatly increased to prevent her combination of physical injury and impaired judgement damaging her further, and someone had to keep a constant eye on her.

For at least four months after coming home from hospital she took the almost total attention of my father and two sisters, who fed, bathed and comforted her. An image of her doing arm-strengthening exercises, hysterical and screaming from pain, will always be in my mind. She would lie in a bed in the glass living-room and weep with pain and frustration and almost from shame – being unable to walk properly or even sit showed a weakness she would never allow. This strength of character is what has driven her recovery, though this same stubbornness has also caused her mental suffering.

Several months passed since the accident before acceptance

really hit me. It was a Saturday night. The family sat in front of a warm, crackly fire to watch a good video. I supported myself with painkillers, a hot-water bottle and pillows, and managed to escape for a brief time and forget that I was now different. Then the video ended and realisation hit me, as if for the first time: 'I am a damaged person, life is not the same.' This realisation opened up another thought: 'I must try to recapture life, I must get back in the world among people.'

Out of My Glass Box
and into the World

My hands trip, my feet trip, my thoughts trip, my tongue trips,
  my brain trips.
I trip therefore I am.

One Saturday morning I asked Ted to take me to a large shopping complex not far from home. I wanted to be out among people again. I quaked and shook, and, feeling like St George off to do battle with the dragon, I carefully walked along the walls of the shops.

It was amazing to be out again, to see so many people and so many children. I had been locked away from the world. How I missed the school and the students. After some time I noticed a little girl looking at me. 'Now, are you from school? Do I know you? Have I taught you?' I asked myself. I smiled at her and she smiled back. It seemed strange and weird – all the children I passed smiled at me, some even craned their necks when they'd passed to smile at me. It wasn't until we passed the Whitmont shirt display that I realised that with my eyepatch they must have thought I was a lady pirate!

This brief glimpse of the world made me desperate to see my students at school again. The trip required a lot of planning. I had to work out when to go and when to get ready.

Out of My Glass Box and into the World

It was a lot of work just to organise a simple visit – only my third out of the home.

The morning of the visit arrived. I remember sitting up in bed howling with pain when the phone on the other side of the bed rang and rang and rang. I couldn't lean across to pick up the receiver, and I was in too much pain to heave myself out of bed to shuffle round to the other side to answer it, so I had no option but to let it ring out.

The dressing (pants, flat shoes and a blouse Ken did up) and getting ready were accomplished. Ken helped me as I gingerly and painfully got into the car. We got to school to find it deserted. Not a pupil or teacher in sight. That unanswered phone call had been from school to say that everyone would be away for the day on an excursion. Later that week we did a repeat of the trip. I did manage to catch up with 'my' kids, a wonderful but painful experience, as they all hugged me.

REHAB: TRAPPED IN A SYSTEM THAT DOESN'T MAKE SENSE

And we all thought 'It couldn't happen to me.
At the Rehabilitation Hospital we all walk funny,
We all talk funny, we all think funny.
But IT'S NOT FUNNY!

Small talk
A bit like a bunch of brides discussing their big day.
But instead of attendants we discussed witnesses,
Instead of clothes the pain,
Instead of the groom, the other party.

Why?
I am innocent
I am innocent
I am innocent
What did I do?

It was now three months since the accident. My GP, Hugh, thought it was time that I went to see a neurologist. Ken and Ann drove me into the city, an amazing surreal world that was familiar, and yet, unfamiliar. Ann walked with me from the car to the building. I fumbled all the way, shaking, afraid, feeling so weird, floaty and different. Was this the same city I had once felt so at home in? I felt an outsider, an interloper in this new world.

Rehab: Trapped in a System that Doesn't Make Sense

The neurologist said I should be assessed for the extent of my head injuries. I was referred to a psychologist at a well-known rehabilitation hospital. On my first visit I completed the tests in a complete daze. I cannot express my horror and amazement when I could not compute simple sums, the sort I had spent hours every week doing with my students. I was given other tests I used to give at school, but I couldn't concentrate long enough to even finish the exercises. I could only just cope, and that was all. Moving and concentrating for short bursts for the intensive testing was very difficult. A week or so earlier it would have been totally impossible.

I began three half-days of rehabilitation a week with occupational therapy, speech therapy, a visit to the psychologist, and private and group balance classes. The program seemed like a sensible way to tackle my problems. I could sleep each afternoon as I was still experiencing extreme exhaustion. On the other two days when I was not at the hospital, I could visit the physio. These visits required a car journey of twenty minutes each way, either with one of the kids driving me, or a taxi ride, a wait, and treatment that was frequently painful. Many times I would sob all the way home in the taxi. What a schedule to stick to! I was exhausted from all the terrifying taxi travel, bewildered from trying to find my way about, and worn out from all the never-ending pain.

I still had no concept of time, and would be full of unreasonable panic, expecting to be late for the appointment. So I would start getting ready at 9 a.m. for the noon arrival of the taxi to take me to the rehabilitation hospital. Ann would help to organise my clothes in the morning, but being alone in the house when the family went off for the day, I had to muddle

Doing Up Buttons

through myself. I would eat lunch at 10 a.m. and be ready for the taxi, then worry why it was late, stumble about the house in fear, and be exhausted when it finally arrived on time. To actually sit in a car required a superhuman effort – I was sure that I would be in another accident. By the time we arrived at the hospital, I would be shaking so much it was hard to walk in the front door.

The moment I stepped into the corridor of the hospital it was as though the filters on my eyes fell off, revealing reality. At home I could stumble, couldn't say what I wanted, repeat myself, and it was just me being a bit strange. But put me in the midst of other head-damaged people and the reason I was the way I was became apparent. Perhaps we have this little antenna inside us that picks up the vibes so we can recognise like people.

The handsome young lawyer wanted to hear from the hoons who'd come over the hill on the wrong side of the road and smashed into his vehicle; the young chap with little face or voice left would weep, wanting to hear from the person who had done this to him; the woman who'd run off the road and into a tree – killing her husband – somehow seemed lucky to have kangaroos to blame!

In the smoke-filled tea-room at the hospital I was interested to hear my query 'Who did this to me?' echoed by so many other people. We must have some innate desire for justice, for those who caused such pain to us to say they're sorry.

Many of my fellow patients were so innocent they made me cry. Some of their stories were so ghastly it was like finding myself suddenly in the middle of a horror movie. To think I had spent my life blissfully unaware that this nightmare world existed.

Snatches of conversation would penetrate my thoughts while I was sitting in the tea-room: 'I got squashed in my car', 'They went through a red light', 'Kangaroos on the road', 'A stolen car chased by police', 'On the wrong side of the road', 'I've been here seven months', 'It happened a year ago', 'Gee, I'm working to talk good!'. My heart bled for all of them. I was appalled at what innocent people in our society have to endure. It was like being whisked to a hell of unimagined misery.

There were so many horrifying stories like Charlie's. He'd been sandwiched between a truck and a tram. He took off his seat-belt to jump clear but realised that he'd land under the tram, so he didn't. Without his seat-belt, he went flying through the windscreen of his car. That was a year ago. All he wanted was to be able to go back to work as a wallpaper hanger. It was apparent — even to me — that he would never be able to do this.

Perhaps the most cruel part of rehab for me was picking up my fellow patients' feelings of fear, pain and hopelessness. Somehow, being aware of the suffering of others so similar to my own, to hear of their obviously unattainable hopes and dreams, made me wonder if I was as unrealistic as them. I shuddered at the thought.

There was the opportunity to observe other patients during group activities and in the tea room. I travelled home in the taxi run with the same people each session, all of us wrapped up in our pain and in our own worlds. I was at the end of the hour-long drop-off journey. One of my fellow travellers had been coming to rehab for five years, which amazed me. I naïvely thought that everyone would be better in that time.

Doing Up Buttons

He'd had his accident on his motorbike. I was even more amazed when, one day on our trip home, he said, 'Good day for a ride. The sun's coming out, there's a bit of wind – freedom. Shame my artificial hip stops me riding.'

The entire rehab experience was so utterly new to me, I had absolutely nothing in my personal experience to relate it to. I felt just like Alice in Wonderland. Did Lewis Carroll write this as an analogy of what it is like to have head injuries? The similarities are too close for comfort! Alice fell down a rabbit hole. She passed many curious things on the way down but was unable to stop to look, or understand what was happening. Alice's fall was down a tunnel towards darkness. There was light at the end of my tunnel. Like Alice, I was shut up inside myself like a folding telescope, in terrifying agony. Thoughts like 'Who am I?' formed in my mind. Like Alice said when she met the caterpillar, 'I'm afraid I can't explain myself, because I'm not myself.' This swearing, unhelpful, pain-racked person who could not see, walk or talk properly, this bumbling idiot child who had to be looked after by her children was not me. I felt wicked. I felt NOBODY understood.

On entering the rehab system I felt I was quite mad. I was thrust into yet another world behind a door in the tunnel of trauma, another world I had not even imagined existed. This world was inhabited by strange people doing and saying crazy things. Through the fog in my mind I could just realise that I resembled these people more than I resembled my 'old' self, my family, friends or past colleagues.

Rehab had its good and bad points. It was very comforting when the doctor showed me the scans of my brain and

Rehab: Trapped in a System that Doesn't Make Sense

pointed out where fluid had drained through the crack in my skull. Seeing proof was so important. A couple of people appeared to understand my condition, they showed empathy and gave me friendship.

I learnt to scan by turning my head from side to side – thus seeing the whole rather than just part of the opening – before going through doorways or going down passages, which helped to reduce the bruising. Rehab gave me a reason to get out of the house and it gave me hope that the experts would fix me. But I found the judgemental approach of all the tests most upsetting. In the past I'd always succeeded in any test I'd attempted, so I was acutely aware of all my numerous lacks and inabilities.

I could not understand the purpose for much that happened to me in rehab. Perhaps the experts tried to explain to me but I couldn't comprehend. I suspect pictures or diagrams would have made more sense than words.

It was also at rehab that I realised you cannot learn from someone who does not appear to like or value you. Some judgements made by the physios were plainly incorrect. For example, a walking stick would have given me so much more confidence. When I inquired about whether a stick would help me, I was told that I was too young to have a stick, and anyway, I would get dependent on a stick and not want to give it up. Five years down the track I say piffle and tosh to the former statement and 'Yes . . . but so what!' to the second. It was only after a couple of years of fumbling about that a physio suggested a stick. The stick has been wonderful for so many reasons: it helps with balance, I have less falls and people don't label me as a drunk.

Doing Up Buttons

One day I actually ganged up with some bikies against the physio. My mates and I were doing some exercises round a tree trunk. The young physio appeared to have no idea how silly, futile and difficult the tasks he was setting us were. If only he had explained what we were doing and why we were doing it! I'd never done anything against authority in my life but his 'them' and 'us' mentality made me rebel. We made fun of him and were quite stupid. Afterwards I felt shocked at myself. I'd behaved badly – I'd disobeyed for the first time in my life – yet I didn't care.

I'd also be overcome by the plight of my fellow patients at unexpected times. Like the time I was sitting in occupational therapy and an eighteen-year-old was wheeled in. We waited together in silence. I said hello and asked him how he was. His answer and the poignancy of the moment shattered me, 'Me smell, me taste, me talk, me thoughts – no good. Me mate, he was on his Ls, he was doing wheelies.' And then he was wheeled away. Several months later I found myself once again waiting with this young guy. He was out of his wheelchair and I commented how good it was that his legs were better. 'Oh, it wasn't me legs,' was his reply. 'It was me head. I'd forgotten how to walk.'

Balance classes were traumatic. Imagine six damaged human beings swaying, faltering and falling, trying to catch a ball. The old man I was throwing the ball to teetered and nearly fell. The young man in the corner eagerly said to the physio, 'See me catch, Coach, I'm doing good, Coach!' The scarred woman in her twenties sat rocking; it was a bad day for her and she kept saying, 'I don't want to be here, I want to go home.'

Rehab: Trapped in a System that Doesn't Make Sense

The same thought sat behind the tears in my head. I looked at them. We all have the 'branding mark': three small puncture scars on our necks from tubes inserted when we were in Intensive Care. I thought, 'If a Martian were to come into the room it might guess that our brains and our balance had been sucked out by some cruel Dracula.'

I worked with greater determination on my balance exercises when I was at home. In the sunshine and with the dog for company I spent hours wobbling my way along the paving cracks in the drive. This was my individual program: I felt some ownership of it, and I wanted to prove something by doing it. This contrasted sharply with trying to fit into a balance group session at the hospital.

I needed lots of explanations and reasons for doing things in rehab. Most of the time I was paralysed with pain and longing for life as it had been. The amazing mental 'trips', the crazy happenings that were wilder than Alice's world were distracting me. When I told the rehab experts they did not appear to understand. I was very disappointed when my mental nonsense was not explained. Later I was to discover it was epilepsy. At the time I felt even more naughty and mad.

Looking back, many things could have assisted me at this stage of my recovery. I desperately needed to talk to someone to help me cope with the loathing and hatred I had of the man who had done this to me. I needed help to deal with the changes in my life, to understand what my husband and family were thinking. I needed to be asked, 'What do you want? What would be most helpful to you?' instead of being judged and told what I needed. Having a say would have empowered me.

Doing Up Buttons

I badly needed a sufferer's manual to help me make sense of the situation, to realise that what I was going through was normal. I needed encouragement rather than the implied criticism I felt from some of the rehab team. Deep down I knew I had a long way to go, so an explanation on why progress would be slow would have been beneficial. I was told that most of my recovery would occur during the first six months, then there would be slow recovery until two years after the accident. Then that would be it.

My GP, Hugh, said he believed that I would continue to improve for five years. I suppose I feel I have made the most helpful progress in recapturing my life in the fifth year. I can remember my panic and consternation as the six-month, then two-year, time barrier passed. The despair I felt that I would be like this for the rest of my life!

I needed help to deal with the loss and grief. I'd lost myself, my ability to be the mother and wife I had been. I'd lost my career, my freedom and my ability to drive. Even shopping for the family's food was an almost impossible task. I needed post-traumatic stress and head damage explained to me, not to be told I was lucky I wasn't more badly hurt or dead.

I didn't want to forget. I needed to try to make sense of this crazy world of rehab and life since the accident, to remember and mourn.

I needed desperately to hear from another Alice who had been down the rabbit hole and survived. I wanted to be told that it was OK to feel frightened and confused. Someone who has sat at the top of the rabbit hole and had a picnic, even if they've peered down, taken photos and studied it, is not as helpful as someone who has fallen down that long, scary hole.

The More You Do the More You See Your Problems

*'Chris, I've told you time and time again not to put gin on your
   weeties in the morning!'*
I've never touched a drop yet I'm 'drunk' all the time!
I've discovered that slower can be faster
I've discovered that frustration can take all my life energy
I've discovered that keeping a diary can let you see progress.

It was now four months since the accident. I struggled and pushed myself to get better – I was absolutely determined to return to school for fourth term. My progress was so slow, like a creeping snail, when before I had done everything at whirlwind pace. At home I wore tracks on the drive doing my walking and balance exercises. I wore out the carpet on the stairs practising stepping up with the right foot, across with the left foot then down with the right foot.

I tried to teach myself the concept of time: everything I did, I timed. I'd guess how long it would take to do something or walk somewhere, then time myself. This was quite difficult because of my problem with numbers – I had lost my one-to-one correspondence. I found an analogue clock much more useful in trying to gauge the passing of time. I could see how much time had passed. I wrote down everything I did, and how long it took me, so I didn't forget. This

Doing Up Buttons

helped me plan a little more efficiently – no longer was I ready at 9 a.m. for a 1 p.m. appointment, instead I'd be ready at 10.30 a.m. From being an invalid who did nothing all day I gradually started to do things again. It was then the breadth and depth of my difficulties became apparent.

I started to be more useful around the house and helped the family by packing and unpacking the top section of the dishwasher on to the bench. I had a smashing time! With the eyepatch on I would ignore my left side and send things flying so they smashed or smashed into other things for double smashings. Without the eyepatch I would put things on the wrong image in the air, again with smashing results. Each week there would be a pile of broken bowls, plates, glasses and vases by the rubbish bin.

My eyes were driving me crazy. I tried patching alternate eyes on alternate days. This meant I'd have days when I couldn't walk straight. It was eerie seeing different colours with each eye, and if I coughed or sneezed in the dark I'd see flashing lights where none existed. Watching television without the patch meant double images: one set on an angle overlapping the other, and once again, the colours differed depending on the eye patched. If I looked at a page of a book with one eye it was green, with the other, cream – which was the real colour?

My eyes had been assessed a week or so after the accident in the hospital and later during a visit to the neurologist. Eventually I was referred to an eye surgeon – the moment I've been waiting for. I'd been patient, I'd waited months for my eyes to settle down, now I could get them fixed. The

The More You Do the More You See Your Problems

surgeon took one look at my pirate patch and said, 'Get that patch off and leave it off – your eyes can't work together if you have a patch. Your eyes have to stop changing.' I stuffed my eyepatch in my pocket and fumbled for the door. Thus started two nightmare months when I went patchless. Down the stairs, falter, fall, double moving images everywhere. My disappointment was great. Now I had to try to survive in this hideous, tilting, moving world.

Unexpectedly and amazingly, my sense of smell returned. I began to depend on touch for my sense of reality. Even the soles of my feet sent me messages. I felt things with my hands – groping things as I passed, embarrassingly, even people. My foot felt or tapped to feel where there were gutters or steps, and I limped as I still couldn't control my left side properly. I walked with my legs far apart, as if I'd just spent a day on a horse. A physio explained that I was doing this automatically to try to get more balance. I felt clumsy, ungainly, ugly and slow. I also experienced sensations of floating. It was all very weird.

Daily the phone calls would come from Mum and Dad. Dad was a great reader and had a deep interest in 'the head' (he'd been a pioneer in the hearing-aid field). He would have numerous suggestions: 'Chick, I've been reading and I think that your fractured orbit is causing a pinched nerve. Paint your glasses with clear nail-polish and when it is nearly dry, smear it. This way your eye can get light, not the darkness behind the patch.' So much love, so much concern and usually an explanation or suggestion that was really useful. Now, five year later, this nail-polished lens is still the most useful thing I've found to deal with the double vision. All the visits to all

Doing Up Buttons

those specialists, and nothing has helped me as much as Dad's suggestion!

My family continued to be saintly and would only occasionally slip out a 'You told us that a second ago.' Ann, Helen and Ken shopped, cooked, cleaned, drove me to countless doctor and hospital appointments and patiently waited with me. They sat with me, tried to cheer me up when I was low, and always had fresh coffee for my visitors. Rob was particularly good at patting me when I wept. Ted hovered around us all, trying to think of anything to alleviate my pain and boredom. From being married to someone who was always interested, busy, happy and full of wonder at the world, he now had a plain, lifeless being who felt no pleasure in anything.

My passion for life had totally melted away. I felt flat and one-dimensional, not the full and multi-dimensional person I had been. I was not a patient patient. Lurking in a hidden part of my brain fluttered the thought 'When I am better, will I be better? Will I ever be better?'

The 'me-I-had-been' loved reading. She dashed off watercolour paintings at a great rate, indeed when living in Mount Isa in Queensland, painting had usurped teaching. She loved nothing better than standing around a campfire when on a school camping trip, squeezing the old piano accordion as the kids' voices leapt to the tall gum trees with the bright sparks of the fire. She loved music, playing piano and guitar, concerts, plays and films, visiting galleries, browsing around the shops with friends or daughters, and eating out. She loved nothing better than getting stuck into the half-acre of garden, mowing and planting – she'd actually slashed much of the hawthorn with a machete while she was pregnant with Ken. When the pool was installed she'd carried two tons of pavers the 150 feet down the hill from the road. This was accomplished within a few days with numerous trips carrying two small pavers wrapped in an old T-shirt.

The country was another passion. Bushwalking, riding the old motorbike, horse and donkey-riding, and mucking around in the country at the family country weekender. Entertaining with the fun and buzz of twenty people for a great breakfast in the sun on the deck. Eating out with the whole family.

Travel, especially off the beaten track, was the *pièce de résistance*. What could be more exciting than exploring Timor in a truck, walking through the rice paddies of Bali, pottering about the back streets of Indonesia in the freshness of dawn with the moon still in the pink sky? Having travelled extensively as a child through Africa, Europe and India, the travel bug was well entrenched. A trip to Europe with the four kids to give them a white Christmas had been a highlight.

This new me was afraid, and shook just to go to the nearby shops in the car.

LORNE

The trip was like a nightmare. The road to Lorne was so
  dangerous.
At first the thought of how long we'd be trapped in the car
When we'd had 'the' accident filled my brain.
Then as we got closer to Lorne the thought
Of the trip in the ambulance scared me witless.
Tomorrow we have to drive home.

Life went on. Ted suggested a short getaway to Lorne. Just two nights away from home, and he believed I'd be a different person. Wow! I really needed to be a different person but there was so much fear to conquer. Just entering the car was a challenge. I knew the chances of being involved in a second accident were slim, but so were the odds of having a first accident, and that had happened.

So it was with my heart in my mouth that we drove first to Queenscliff. Sitting beside a roaring fire in a room full to overflowing with luscious bowls of flowers I felt the nightmare shimmer and shift. The pain was still as ghastly, and I needed an afternoon nap, but subtly I was starting to feel some awakening that I might be a 'real' person again.

Before dinner we took a stroll along the pier and around the town. Even though I had to feel the way, touching trees, fences and railings to get my bearings, I could feel the calm and beauty of the evening. Dinner was superb and I only knocked my knife off the table once and spilt only a little food. Things were indeed looking up. We had a cheery fire glowing in our room when we went upstairs, and I felt the shadow of happiness flowing in my veins for the first time in months.

Unfortunately and unbelievably, I awoke at midnight shaking with pain and the most violent gastric attack I'd ever suffered, and ended up spending the night in the quaint bathroom across the hall. Weeks and tests later confirmed that I'd picked up a nasty bug in hospital. Why it chose that night to rear its ugly head I'll never know. After a squeamish breakfast in the delightful breakfast room came another big decision: to stay another night in Queenscliff or to drive on to Lorne. My inclination was to stay another night, but Ted had a passion to go further down the coast.

We got to Lorne and Ted helped me into the room, brought in our belongings and then sat me on the patio with the view of the sea and coastline stretching out in front of us. He then left me and went into the township. When he'd gone, I howled. Was this just a reaction to the dangerous drive? Or was it the double wavy horizon making me sick? Or was it a longing to be as I was this time last year, when we'd bounded down to town for a coffee, full of happiness? In anger and frustration I left the patio and threw myself down on the motel bed, badly miscalculating distance and banging my head violently on the bed-head. When I opened my eyes I was bitterly disappointed. I still couldn't see properly, the way characters can in cartoons.

Ted returned, proudly sporting ten red tulips in a borrowed

vase. Five months earlier, when we had been in New York, Ted had bought me ten pink tulips and put them in a milk carton. Same sentiment, same flowers, same number, same Ted. But a different country, different colours, different containers and a different me. Weeping, I removed the eyepatch and there were twice as many flowers, twice the sentiment and twice the gratitude.

Ted said he'd give his right arm or ten years of his life to take away my pain. Just knowing of the offer made the pain more bearable. It's strange that for four months we'd been unable to discuss how we really felt about the accident. I had felt Ted's anger and now, years later, can recognise it for what it was – anger at the man who did this to me, the person who had changed our lives. At the time I felt so different, ungainly, out of control, stupid and unlovable, I secretly thought he must be angry at me for wrecking our lives.

Sitting at a table in the fish-and-chip shop, biting into a piece of flake, Ted said he was so glad to see a shine back in my unpatched eye. He spoke of sad nights at dinner when my lifeless eye nearly broke his heart. He said he loved me. How could he? I felt so completely unlovable. I was desperately searching for proof. Foolishly, I thought, 'If he loved me he would have got me out of the hell of that six-bed ward.' And yet I knew he'd believed that I was in the best place. He appeared to become angry when I wept, when in fact he was upset and frustrated that he could not help me. We had been married for twenty-five years and had always shared our hopes and beliefs and fears. But without any experience of this situation, and with no counselling, how were we to know how to tackle things?

Lorne

Once Ted was able to pat me when I cried, I felt a lot better. He'd exclaim, 'Patting you can't make you better!' It did. He wanted to do something practical to make things better. He somehow blamed himself that I had had the accident, as if it was his task in life to protect me, and he had failed. He wanted to fix the problems – to send me to another specialist, put more cushions behind me, get me a painkiller – when all I wanted from him was a pat! But all our energies were directed at trying to make life seem as normal as quickly as possible for the kids. We were playing the game that life was still the same. Now we had both the time and inclination to start bringing out some of our fears and hopes into the open.

Taxi-drivers who did the rehabilitation run would tell me that the saddest part about accidents was how they break up marriages, or, as one driver put it, 'The tiniest hairline crack would widen and split them apart.' I suppose our trip to Lorne was like super-glue.

When we returned home I wrote: 'I think I'm starting to feel a little better. Today I saw two small girls, Brownies, sitting on a fence. There was a woman peeping through the blinds at her new front fence. I could feel her glee and happiness. A black dog with white socks was trotting through the gate after his master – faithfulness and warm fur – wonderful animals.' It's funny that I haven't seen scenes like this for months.

Uni: Trying to Find 'Me'

I've discovered that we only see what we look at.
I've discovered that it's hard to know where to look.
I've discovered that it's hard to understand what you see.

I had a one-track mind. I decided that if I could get back to uni and work on my Master's degree, I would find the 'old' me. I just had to try to do it. After much soul-searching and working out of practicalities – who would take me and pick me up – we all decided that I should try to continue my degree. In a way, all of us felt that my pain and suffering would all have been in vain if I gave up. Somehow, to continue seemed a positive, active step in thwarting The-Man-who-had-hit-me, preventing him from ruining my life.

In hindsight my first night of lectures alone was crazy! The trip in to uni terrified me. Ted took me, helped me find the lecture room, sat me in a seat and, bless his heart, stayed and took notes for me. Ken, Helen and Ann each volunteered to accompany and help me.

The subject was a continuation of the Futures in Education course I had completed in a summer school at the beginning of the year. There was a weekly two-hour evening lecture. Rick, the lecturer, was most supportive and helpful. My peers were kind. At first it felt as if the lecture was conducted in a

Uni: Trying to Find 'Me'

foreign language — I certainly could not understand a word of what he was saying.

Rick ran the classes by giving notes to read at home before the lecture. The kids read them to me, but they made no sense. After several weeks of perseverance and discussions with Ken and Helen about the topic, I started to understand a little. Ted increased the size of the type of the notes, and I used a ruler and finger to slowly follow each line and repeated the facts out loud. Gradually I understood fragments of what Rick was talking about. How excited I felt when I could grasp the meaning of a sentence! This was working. By working hard I was convinced I could improve. Slowly, slowly I could try to recapture this section of my life.

The subject I was taking was a sequel to one I had taken just before the accident. This meant that the content and much of the terminology were familiar. In the past I'd typed all my projects but the boys felt a computer would help. It did. The computer meant that I could slowly make notes in big print. It became possible for ideas to come out via my fingers on the keyboard when it would have been hard to say or read the words.

It was so interesting — I could not understand a novel but to study a familiar subject was possible with heaps of help and encouragement from my family. At times I would record ideas on to a tape as I lay in bed and the kids would type them up. Study certainly provided an activity I could do at my own pace when I felt well enough. Even if it was just ten minutes a day, I felt as if I was achieving something. If I had time to spend waiting for an appointment with the physio or the

Doing Up Buttons

doctor, I'd pull out a page or two of notes and a marker.

Tutorials were another thing altogether. They were a huge challenge because I had such trouble reading out loud and my memory was so poor. I could have read the same paragraph over and over again and not realised I'd just read it. Placing my finger on each word helped, but was rather slow and ungainly for presenting a uni paper. So I found things that could become my cues and help me to speak. I thought of using several different boxes or chests with matches or chess pieces in them to get the message across. Pictures and symbols and charts written by Ann spoke to me and my audience more than words. Of course, this meant that Ken or Ann had to get me and my bag of tricks to and from uni.

Uni was a wonderful measure with which to gauge my progress. We graduated from Ted having to take me by the hand to physically put me in a chair and a pencil in my hand, to Ken supporting my weight as we fumbled our way to the lecture, to Ann leading me across the road. Then came the day when she waited and watched in the car, heart in her mouth, while I crossed the road on my own. Later she said she felt just as I must have as I watched her learn to cross the road at primary school. Talk about role reversal!

Nowadays I would be the one to make the house untidy and the kids would pick up after me. Ann would still put out my clothes because I didn't know what kind of clothes I liked or which shirt went with what pants or jacket. Ann was a great help when it came to getting dressed. She seemed to forever be saying: 'Oh Mum, you can't go out looking like that! Come here and I will do up your buttons in the right holes!'

Uni: Trying to Find 'Me'

One day Ann took me to a large shopping complex to help me move about among people. I decided I wanted a pie for lunch. Admittedly it's years since I've tried to eat a pie out of a paper bag, but within one second I was covered in pie and couldn't even begin to figure out what to do, so I just went on trying to eat the pie. It didn't occur to me to try to wipe up the mess. Ann disappeared, I panicked. When she reappeared clutching a handful of paper serviettes, I still didn't understand what was going on. So Ann carefully cleaned me up and led me to the car.

It's amazing that I, mother of four, teacher of five-hundred, wiper-up extraordinaire of messes, foreseer of potential messes, was so lost, so powerless.

School: Trying to Find 'Me' (ii)

I've discovered that doing something useful helps you feel good about yourself

I've discovered that my concept of who I am is tied up with what I do

I've discovered that the more you try to forget something the more you will remember.

I've discovered that the more you try to remember something the more you will forget.

In order to recapture my old life I felt I had to return to school, to teaching. 'How could you teach?' I hear you ask. That I even contemplated such a thing is an example of how muddled my thinking was. I was still experiencing horrific pain, and my ribs poked out like a bird's wing in my back. My left leg dragged, and this brought on unbelievable muscle pain; indeed frequently I could not walk when I first woke up and would have to crawl upstairs in the morning. My left hand was clenched, my palm would be marked by my nails.

I was suffering from fatigue so I only had a couple of 'good' hours a day. I had double vision, I was blacking out momentarily and all in all, I was still in a very bad way. Mentally I was hopeless. I could not remember things. My sense of time, space and ideas of numbers had gone. Yet I was totally

School: Trying to Find 'Me' (ii)

insistent that I get back to school. It really was too early in my recovery, but I was adamant.

School meant so much to me: the students, my colleagues, the ideas – it was my life. I just couldn't imagine life without teaching. Every day since I left hospital I'd thought, 'When I get back to school, life will be right.'

Fran, the understanding person from rehab, was there to assist me to find my way back to work. She was there to protect me from failing, to be supportive and pick up the pieces when the going got tough. It was her task to analyse the job requirements and to try to match my skills to the job. She also had to make sure I was not a danger to myself or others. She had to explain to the Head of the school that people who suffered from acquired brain damage may display the following difficulties: fatigue, difficulty in concentration and loss of memory. She did not list all my deficits as she felt that doing so would only make them more obvious.

No-one knew what progress I would make. To be truthful, not one of the specialists believed that I would be able to return to full-time teaching. Of course this was just a red rag to a bull, and made me even more determined to do so and prove them all wrong. Notwithstanding every ounce of effort I have put into getting better, I must now admit they were right, but I wasn't to know this at the time. Indeed, if I had known that five years later I would only be able to work two mornings a week, I would have totally given up and wallowed in despair.

After many lengthy discussions between the school, the doctors, the hospital and Fran, it was decided that I was not yet ready to return to my grade six girls. I was absolutely shattered. I had tried so hard to get better and I'd failed. I felt

Doing Up Buttons

I'd not only failed myself, but also my family and my school, and last, but not least, my pupils and their families. My pupils had kept regular contact with me in the expectation I would return to be their teacher in fourth term. I tried to explain the situation to them by writing a letter to each of them, to go with a made-up 'Rehab Report'.

REHABILITATION REPORT ON CHRIS DURHAM

1. Walking – Balance – Eyesight

Chris is learning to scan where she is going before she walks through doorways. This skill is reducing damage both to door frames and her arms. She is trying hard with her balance exercises and is of less danger to herself and others.

She is learning to monitor herself when she feels she is 'floating'. As she still has a lot of trouble judging distance and depth, we recommend she takes out a new insurance policy to cover breakages.

Chris should make sure there isn't a car in sight when she steps out on to the road, even though she is learning new vocabulary from people driving the cars she walks in front of. When pouring a cup of coffee, a finger in the mug to judge depth will save wiping up spills.

2. Talking

Chris is finding ways of coping when she a) forgets words; b) makes up strange words; c) forgets what she is talking about; and d) forgets what you are talking about.

3. Shopping

Chris must take greater care not to queue-jump through not scanning properly, as this tends to cause awkward moments. She must also take more care when walking near large stacks of cans – this can cause even more difficult moments.

4. Other
More work still needs to be put into doing up buttons, not dropping things or knocking over vases, people or cups, and not stepping on dogs or cats.

5. Homework
Chris must learn to slow down and rest for ten minutes each hour.

How could I explain double vision to the kids? I wrote 'Chris's Song', to be sung to the last verse of 'The Twelve Days of Christmas'.

> When I get up each morning this is what I see ... two right hands, two cheery husbands, two black dogs, two cakes of soap ... two shiny toasters ... two bowls of flowers, two Helens, two Kens, two Anns and two tall Robs. And then I put my eyepatch on!

It was decided that I would return to school for a couple of mornings a week to do alternative duties. I was to be a 'useful person', listing equipment in the science and maths store rooms, and helping in the library, covering books and so on. After several weeks of this regime I was to take a half-hour philosophy and discussion session as enrichment or extension with a group of five girls. After a couple more weeks I would take two small group classes, widely interspersed with my library work.

Doing Up Buttons

I must confess my first morning at school was a bit of a disaster. For a start the kids all wanted to hug me, which was a trifle painful, but it was wonderful to be with the kids and my colleagues, to catch up on their news, and to feel part of the school again. But there was the strange sensation of not belonging, of not having a spot to call your own. Although I still had a passionate interest in the kids from my grade, they were no longer 'mine'. In fairness to them and their new teacher, I had to let them go.

I started cataloguing the science equipment, weeping silently into my eyepatch. Let me tell you, a soggy eyepatch is no fun. I badly wanted to be useful, but it took so long for me to understand or do things. Tasks that before would have been done in a flash now required amazing concentration, not only to grasp what the task was, but to remember what I was doing. I seemed to have incredible difficulty with concepts, ideas and even remembering why I was at school but not in my classroom. I was constantly having to say to myself, 'I've had an accident – that's why I'm doing this.'

The library was my salvation – a bottomless pit of new books to process and labels to stick. The concentration required was perfect rehabilitation: teaching my hands to obey me, relearning the alphabet, struggling with the double vision. I was very fortunate that the school supported me as they did. They must have had a great deal of concern about what sort of legal liability I would present were I to fall!

After several weeks I started working with one group, then two groups, each of five girls, for half an hour each morning, discussing philosophy. This was both wonderful and terrible. I had great difficulty planning the half-hour sessions, so I used

School: Trying to Find 'Me' (ii)

work that I'd written up before the accident. What amazing discussions we had, but how frustrating as well! No matter what I did, I couldn't remember a name or what we were talking about a minute after we'd discussed something.

Was this progress? It was exciting to be a 'teacher' again, but somehow I knew I was not the same teacher I had been.

As the year drew to a close, my hopes that I would be who I was faded. As my general well-being improved, I gained a greater understanding of my problems.

When I was not taking philosophy sessions I continued my struggle with helping in the library. The students were magnificent. I've never had any discipline problems, apart from the students getting a little loud in their enthusiasm; they were kind, tolerant, friendly, interested and understanding. I attribute much of my satisfaction and happiness to the wonderful support of the girls.

In order to follow our discussions I would make notes on a large sheet of paper. My spelling had gone the same way as my maths. The students kindly helped me by correcting my work. I had quite a bit of trouble writing as I had forgotten the alphabet, and would put unrelated letters in words. In the older groups one student or another would say, 'Don't worry, we'll write for you.' It's most humbling to have a student take the Texta from your fingers to take over the role of recorder.

The new Preps would think I was a pirate lady or that I had no eye beneath the patch, but once I had shown them my eye they accepted it, and only occasionally needed to check – just to make certain it was still there. I hope I didn't cause nightmares of the one-eyed lady!

Helen and Ann started a collection of walking sticks with

different heads for me. The students loved to open one stick with the compass and flask; they patted the duck head or horse's head that formed a handle on the other sticks. Occasionally I would come across a group of girls 'playing philosophy', having very meaningful conversations with the leader needing a stick (a blackboard ruler usually worked well). My stick seemed to be constantly in demand as a prop for plays; so much so that I kept a spare at school to lend to the girls who needed it.

Over the next few years I would be overwhelmed with frustration and guilt because no matter how hard I tried, I could not remember students' names. I tried making cardboard name labels to place in front of each student. This was a dismal failure as they all tended to play with them or, worse still, bang them on the table, trying my double vision and sensitive hearing. My patience and coping strategies were very poor in such circumstances. Then I tried using colour-coded name labels with a loop of different coloured ribbons to place round a top button on their school uniform – not the most dignified thing for the girls. Then I asked them to bring a pin or plastic name tag from home – also not a good idea. I tried getting them to write their names on the page they were working on, but that did not solve my problem. It was quite frightening to realise that many of us judge someone's values and determine if we like someone by whether or not that someone can be bothered to remember our name. It took me two years of frustration, shame and anger before I came up with a solution to my name problem. Wool.

As a part of my school program, I developed a lesson whereby we used wool as a symbol of a discussion model.

School: Trying to Find 'Me' (ii)

We threw the wool across the table to indicate how everybody gets a turn to speak. I then got the students to place the tangled wool on the table and asked them what it looked like.

Someone would say, 'a spider's web'.

'What's a web for?' I would ask.

'To trap food', would be the reply. Then I'd explain that I forgot things, and how sometimes we all had difficulty remembering things, and needed a trap for our thoughts – a 'thinking trap'. So our philosophy journals would be called 'Thinking Traps'.

After starting a discussion I would throw the messy ball of wool to someone with their hand up to start the discussion. They would then throw the ball of wool to someone who wanted to add a point. Possession of the wool meant they had the floor. Names were no longer crucial. The students ran the discussions themselves and the most amazing spin-off was that pulling and playing with the wool seemed to loosen tongues and thoughts.

It was also a non-threatening way to stop certain students from hogging the discussion. It was much easier to say, 'You've had the wool several times' instead of 'You talk all the time'. The girls are now 'programmed', like Pavlov's dogs, so that when they get the wool in their hands they often talk from notes they've been scribbling in their journals. A couple of times a lesson I'd ask them to pass the wool around so that everyone, even the very shy, contributes to the discussion.

I must confess this wool business has led to some quite crazy episodes, like the time several girls were 'busting' with ideas only to be told in a superior way by the person speaking 'I've got the wool, so listen to me!' It's quite a spectacle, I tell you! Not to be beaten, the frustrated speaker-to-be's beady eye

Doing Up Buttons

spied a scrap of red wool on a shelf (we shared our room with Craft). The speaker quickly retorted, 'No! It's got to be a ball of red wool!' Like lightning the other lass rubbed her hands together, rolling the scrap into a minute ball which she displayed to us between her fingertips. As you can imagine by this time we were all rolling round the floor, laughing, but we quietened down enough for her to put forward her point.

By giving each student a cent we would describe and discuss cents, scents and sense. Another session was based on a can of baked beans. I asked 'What fairy story has the word beans in it?' 'Jack and the Beanstalk,' was the reply. We then discussed if Jack was good or bad, giving reasons for the statements. Little Preppies would ask, 'Was Jack good to kill the bad giant?', 'Is it good to kill a bad person?' and 'How do we know if someone is good or bad?' Some day I will write of the thinking adventures we have had.

It felt so strange to be standing at the school gate at noon, waiting for the taxi that would take me home. On arriving home I would fall into bed and sleep soundly for several hours, frequently waking so deathly cold it was frightening. I'd manage somehow to stiffly struggle to the shower and stand under near-boiling water for up to twenty minutes, but I would still feel frozen to the bone. My head damage meant that my body didn't control my temperature.

Then it would be time to psych myself up to appear normal when the family arrived home. What a life! What a waste of a life!

During this time I'd gone patchless for a couple of months. Then I was told by the same specialist to put my patch back on. The complexity of my double vision was

School: Trying to Find 'Me' (ii)

starting to emerge as my eyes settled down. Apparently both eyes were twisted from the horizontal and vertical planes, which meant I did not see the ground as level with either eye. I had hoped surgery could straighten up one eye to the other, but according to the specialist, both eyes had to be moved. Several operations to each eye were discussed. There was also a likelihood that the eyes would revert to how they were. My eye-surgeon referred me to yet another specialist, but he was not keen to operate yet. More time was needed for my eyes to settle.

I was absolutely devastated. My plans of returning to school to take grade six the following year were dashed. The bitterest blow of the year was accepting the advice of the medicos that I would not be fit for full-time duties for some time.

Thinking back on it all, I can remember my totally dogged determination that 'Yes, I can teach next year' when all the evidence to hand indicated that I would not be able to cope. I can't describe the sadness and despair I felt as Ted helped me move my gear from my classroom. Would I ever have my own class again? Would I ever use all my charts and pictures and books again? I wept as we placed all my stuff in boxes and Ted carted them to the school attic. I just hoped that I would be needing them again.

Discussions were held with Fran from rehab and Phillipa, the Head of the school. It was decided that I was to work teaching philosophy interspersed with making myself useful in the library. How fortunate I was to belong to such a caring workplace. How fortunate I was that they would give me alternative duties while I continued down the long road to recovery.

Reality and Unreality Clash

In the blink of an eye
I am in that surreal other world
That strange world
The 7th dimension, virtual reality,
Where unreality is more real than reality.

1991 drew to a close. Now six months after the accident, I would find myself on the most amazing, surreal trips. I would be calmly doing something, like biting into a cherry, when suddenly I would find myself a twelve-year-old, sitting in a tree with my brother. These trips were more vivid than reality, brighter than technicolour. They were like the nightmares I had experienced in hospital.

At other times I'd detect a pungent burning smell. So frequently did these things happen that I started to believe I was going mad. It was too difficult to explain, too weird. It was my terrible secret.

On one of my numerous visits to the neurologist she remarked that I had damage to the area of my brain that epileptics have damaged. She asked me if I was having epileptic fits. 'Oh no,' I answered with surety. I'd had teacher training. I knew that an epileptic fit was when you lay on the floor with a ruler in your teeth. I didn't think to report that when I first came round in Intensive Care I discovered I'd

Reality and Unreality Clash

bitten a large chunk off my tongue. I think I did mention how it drove me crazy that I was frequently nipping my tongue with my teeth. This hurt so much it would constantly wake me up.

Early in the new year these issues came up once more. Again I tried to voice my blanking-out episodes. This time I received an explanation for my trips: epilepsy. I wasn't going mad. Relief washed over me.

I was prescribed Tegretol. The effect of the drugs was wonderful. I could think with greater clarity, make connections and links. Somehow messages seemed to get through. I felt almost normal. Three weeks later though, I felt really odd.

One Sunday morning Ted took me to the doctor. 'I don't know what's wrong, but my whole body feels out of control ... I'm scared ... could I be having a reaction to the drugs?' Unfortunately Hugh wasn't on that morning and the doctor and I got side-tracked discussing chest infections and other things. (Chest infections hovered about me, and the possibility of having an infection was always there. I subsequently learnt from specialists in New York that this is common with head injury.)

Antibiotics were prescribed. In the following days I returned to the doctor. The antibiotics were changed. A week passed. I lay in my glass room, moaning. I became sicker and sicker. I could only eat boiled potatoes, and I had a fever and terrible pains in my joints day and night. My heart felt as if it was squashed by an elephant. I could walk no more than a couple of steps at a time. Another week, and tests indicated possible hepatitis and trouble with my heart. We waited days to find out what sort of hepatitis it was. Throughout this

Doing Up Buttons

trauma, my only aim in life was to eat a potato so that I wouldn't take my epilepsy drugs on an empty stomach. I writhed on my bed. I was sure I was dying. When I started to vomit up white soapy stuff, my mind flashed to the story of Madame Bovary and how she died after taking poison. 'I'm poisoned', I told myself. And indeed I was – it was a violent reaction to the epilepsy drug.

I stopped taking the medication. As my heart was affected it seemed safer to try to manage with no medication. Gradually the seizures became less frequent, and compared with several a day during the first three years after the accident, I now may experience only one blanking-out a week.

END OF THE YEAR WHEN MY LIFE CHANGED

I've planted punnet after punnet of seedlings.
I've just realised that to me they're a talisman, a symbol
That come Christmas they'll flower into a facsimile of the flower on the label,
And I hope that come Christmas I'll flower too
That I'll flower into my old self.

I was still experiencing difficulty trying to appear normal. The way I walked and talked made me appear as if I was a little drunk all the time. I certainly needed to be less sensitive about the way people would take a step back and watch my ungainly gait as I tried to feel my way about. I felt very much a 'lesser person' when people would retreat from me as I struggled to find the post and the pedestrian lights on my way to a doctor's appointment in the city.

I also needed to be very careful when trying to cross the road or railway line near school. One morning I ran in front of an oncoming train because I couldn't recognise what it was. I saw the barrier go down and thought I was a child in a race. I just ran across the train tracks with my stick and bag of school books.

I had to try to remember to only cross the road at traffic lights. With visual inattention and poor visuo-spatial ability,

Doing Up Buttons

I'd become lost at supermarkets, at school and at home. I felt so confused and frightened, upset and stupid when mis-seeing things.

Tears of frustration and sadness would spring out of my eyes when I forgot words. I was starting to become an expert at pretending that I understood what was going on or what people said, but there had been little or no improvement in my comprehension at all. Due to receptive dysphasia I have difficulty in understanding the meanings of words I do not know or do not understand. At school, my day-to-day forgetfulness made conversations with the staff a difficulty. Most of the time I was confused and bewildered, and unable to initiate an important conversation with Ted or at school without making notes first. At times, when I was faced with a task that I couldn't grasp, I was full of overwhelming dread and fear. I was afraid that I was no longer in control of situations and this exacerbated my anxiety, and led to a growing tendency to withdraw from social contact.

It felt so silly to have to make notes to have a discussion with Ted. I must also have been an incredibly irritating person to have a discussion with, because I had to say what I wanted to say when I thought of it, or else I'd lose my thought. This meant I had to interrupt people when they were speaking or make notes. After some time I realised that I needed to know the topic people were talking about before I could understand what they were saying or make links in my head. It's amazing how often in conversation the explanation or punch line is left until the last moment. Ted might be in full flight telling me something and I'd need to stop him. I'd ask him to explain how what he was saying fits into what we have been discussing.

End of the Year When My Life Changed

I was also plagued by a partial disregard of common-sense and judgement. My frontal-lobe damage meant it was difficult to control emotions, and behave appropriately. I later learnt that this was the reason I was too familiar with strangers and frequently said inappropriate, 'silly' things.

As the end of the year approached, changes were afoot. Helen obtained vacation work in Thailand, so she went off for four months to work in a large law firm in Bangkok. We had gone to live in Thailand when she was in grade six and all the kids but Rob had attended the International School there. Rob had clung to my knees as I studied for a Bachelor of Education by correspondence at home in the comparative cool of the mornings. The kids would arrive home at lunchtime, school over for the day, and we would spend the afternoons together. Weekends would be spent exploring or at the British Club. We'd all loved the sights, sounds and smells of Asia.

Helen's boyfriend, Greg, went to Thailand to join her and they returned home happy and engaged. We were all thrilled. Greg had been so much a part of the family for several years. A musician, his song, written to wish Helen a happy birthday on her twenty-first birthday, became a big hit.

Helen's move to Thailand allowed Ann to move into Helen's room in a student house. Suddenly I'd lost two supporters. Life was not going to be as pleasant. I could not help but feel that Ann must have been secretly relieved to leave home and my dependency on her. I was glad she would have some freedom, but sad to lose her company and help. She would still come home to cook, shop or clean up, but I felt lost without my 'live-in' companion. I was now completely

Doing Up Buttons

dependent on the boys: Ken, who was continuing with his Arts degree and Rob, who was in Year Ten at school.

In December we had a CCC open house. The invitation asked our guests to say 'Si Si', to join in an afternoon of celebration: Ted and kids had survived so far, Helen was off to Bangkok, Chris was starting to feel a little better; conviviality and coffee. To have friends, helpers and family with us was so good.

The year my life changed was drawing to a close, and soon it was Christmas. That morning we woke up to the sound of carols floating up the valley from the park where the local band plays an annual dawn concert. Marcus and his family cooked Christmas dinner for the clan. How wonderful to belong to a close family. As I rested in the glass-room I tried to find a way of expressing how I felt as the year ended. The flutter of a bird's wing caught my eye. That's it, I thought! The story of the birds and my one 'late bloomer' tells how I felt.

I think it was early summer when they made their first visit. Mum, Dad and the four babies. From my bed in the glass-room overlooking the valley, I watched with interest as the new family paid a visit to the bird feeding-tray in a nearby tree. My slow and painful recovery had been cheered by the daily visits of my many feathered friends. The seasons passed and the birds changed with them. The curlews, the wild doves that cooed as they ruffled their pinkish breasts, and four kookaburras hung around until I scrounged some meat for them (at the worst, tinned dog food), and now the faithful magpies had retuned for yet another season of feeding and singing for their supper, or at least delighting us with their antics to repay us for providing them with a restaurant.

End of the Year When My Life Changed

From the first day my eye was caught by one of the babies. This bird was smaller than the other babies and perched in the tree, watching with its beady eyes as its greedy siblings were fed by the parents.

It made twice the noise of the others and frequently appeared to miss out entirely on being fed because it was so busy squawking. Weeks and months passed till the babies were as large as their parents. I would watch with interest as the babies would clamour to be fed by their poor parents. I suppose our kids are as tall, if not taller than us, and they still need us to provide the food!

By this time I felt quite distressed by my 'slow one', as I'd called him. I'd noticed that, like me, he had great trouble balancing to walk, he stumbled and at times missed the branch or feeding-tray when he landed. I would try to put out two lots of food, hoping he would be able to feed in peace, but the others would quickly tackle the new pile of food. By now I was sure that the scrawny, noisy bird would perish.

But I started to notice a skinny, lone visitor at odd times, calling to me to replenish the food in the tray. I watched with amazement as he negotiated and manoeuvred himself to pick up the oats his family had spilt during their feeding frenzy. Yesterday as I went to the laundry door, there was a plump sleek maggie sifting through the scraps – my 'slow one' – the only one from the family of six to realise that just round the corner was a constant supply of scraps. He is still a little clumsy at times and hangs back from the crowd, but he has his own way of coping and getting by.

It looks as if I'd be better off to look to the back door of life to give me my opportunities.

In Court

Dancing with the Lawyer for the Defence.
I was put in an excruciating position today.
I could think and feel outrage for the way you were 'playing' with my emotions
Deep inside my head warning bells were ringing
I knew you were trying to trap me yet I could not process or comprehend
I certainly could not follow your dance step
As you kept changing the tune.

One Saturday morning Ted took me to the police station to make a statement. The young police officer allowed me time to try to put together my statement. He spoke of holding the intravenous drip for me as I was being attended to by the ambulance crew. He said how he felt frustrated with the man who had hit me because he appeared so indifferent and uncaring. In chatting after we had completed the paper work, he said his sister had gone to Ivanhoe Girls' Grammar. When he repeated his surname I realised that I had taught her. It's a small world.

In the new year I was subpoenaed to be a witness in the Criminal Court. At this stage of my recovery I was still in considerable pain. I had difficulty walking, and my thinking and reasoning were slow and laborious. I had difficulty

In Court

grasping the meanings of conversations, and speaking was a huge effort. We called into the police station to meet the police officer prosecuting the case; he told me to relax and just tell the truth. The police charged Mr X with dangerous driving, failing to stop at a stop sign and failing to render assistance.

I was to appear as a witness on the first day of court. Ted and I sat outside the courtroom, waiting. It was a thrill to see Peter, who had saved my life, but I felt so guilty that he had to miss work because of my case. A stranger came up and introduced himself to me, and so I learnt of how Steve, a passing tow-truck driver, had helped Peter smash the passenger-side window to break into the car and take off the choking seat-belt. I suppose it was inappropriate behaviour, but he knelt before me while I sat on the bench in the busy court waiting-room. We held hands and beamed at each other.

Another man was sitting on another bench. That had to be the despised Mr X. I was amazed that my fury, anger and hurt had vanished. In their place were sympathy and compassion.

I was called into court. The door opened and I was swallowed up in a room with no windows. I was overcome with claustrophobia. Panic surfaced. All I could think was that I was only a few seats from the man who had ruined my life. I wanted to scream and shout, to point at him and say, 'Look what you've done!'

The police had done a trade-off with the other side – they would drop the 'failing to stop at a stop sign' charge if the lawyer from the other side would be 'gentle with me'. However, I had to remain silent and listen to his lawyer explain that it was all *my* fault. You could have knocked me

Doing Up Buttons

over with a feather when this bit of information finally managed to filter through into my mind.

Once I took the stand his lawyer asked me if I would be too upset to look at a photo of the street where the accident occurred. My mind did a hiccup. What? It was not the road that nearly killed me, it was that man! My mind was in a furious whirlwind.

He showed me a photo of the accident site with large trucks parked along the road. 'He only poked the front of his car out to see past the trucks.'

I couldn't comprehend – there were no trucks there, it was a no parking zone. I was so sure the world had gone mad. It had all seemed so obvious, so simple, that I just couldn't believe my ears and mind. I could hardly follow the crazy ideas that were being put forward. Then it was suggested I was speeding because I was in a hurry.

From the recesses of my mind floated the fact that I was early that day. I can't remember if the right words came out of my mouth.

The pain in my back felt like a chainsaw. The world was whirling around me. In the end I could only manage two hours in court. Ted took me home during lunchtime and put me to bed, and then returned for the rest of the sitting.

There were another two days of court but there was no way I could have attended on those days, or coped. Ted and my parents attended the sittings, which were spread out over the period of a month. Ted would return home after each day in court to inform me of the proceedings. Of how Mr X would say how he smashed the window to turn off the ignition and Peter would explain that the driver's window was down so he

In Court

just had to put his hand in the window to turn off the ignition. It became a battle between Mr X and Peter. Apparently Peter was superb (according to the police, the best witness they'd ever had). At last Mr X was found guilty of dangerous driving and failing to render assistance. His punishment was a fine of one thousand dollars and two years off the road.

In some strange way, having my day in court helped me to come to terms with having the accident. It was almost as if the hearing was an acknowledgment of the event. The accident had occurred. My life had changed. It was good to let go and stop focusing on Mr X, and to try to get on with the rest of our lives.

The next episode came from our insurance company. Mr X was claiming that I was partly responsible for the accident so once again, we were on the court merry-go-round.

At this time I was very ill – as it turned out, a reaction to the anti-epilepsy drug. I could not eat, I shook, my heart felt as if it was tearing out of my body, I could hardly walk and I had to go to court. Also, I was terrified after the last time. We met the barrister from the insurance company at the accident scene early in the morning. Ted showed him the street as I lay shaking in the car. We then drove to court. I was so ill I couldn't get out of the car so Ted left me lying on the back seat and went to find out when I was needed so he could come to get me. I suppose he would have had to half carry me into the courtroom. After waiting for what seemed an eternity he returned to the car, leapt into the driver's seat and started the engine. He was taking me home to bed. Mr X's insurance company had admitted liability on the courthouse steps.

Relief at Mr X's admission of liability was both profound and gratifying. It was one thing that went right, one thing that made sense.

Once the first criminal case established that I was not responsible, I could start the long process of being assessed by doctors for the civil action. But the next few months proved that I was still like a puppet, powerless in a crazy world where I was forced by others to obey commands. This sensation of powerlessness continued through the round of doctors to prove that I was more than 30 per cent incapacitated. These doctors' visits were on top of the eight doctors I had visited to be assessed for Workcare and Transport Accident Commission requirements.

A letter advising me to attend a series of doctors' appointments at various widespread locations soon arrived. Costs for taxis to these medical appointments, as well as the consultations, were to be covered by the Transport Accident Commission. The visits were like some sort of macabre lucky dip. As each doctor was to write a report on my condition, the consultations were frequently long and laborious. It was traumatic finding my way around by taxi, locating the doctor's rooms in the maze of hospital corridors and arriving on time in my bewildered, dazed state. On more than one occasion I was treated unkindly. The inference appeared to be that I was a nuisance, a cheat and a liar. Rarely did I feel like a human being after a session where I was yelled at to bend or move. Sometimes tests would be repeated many times, until the doctor could prove I really was capable of doing something; never mind that these results had been achieved by causing great pain and suffering.

In Court

At times, especially with tests where you had to put blocks or patterns together, the doctor would place the puzzle together, then push the pieces a quarter of an inch out and ask me to complete the test. If I had coached my students as well for tests, they would have all come out geniuses!

One day I had to visit both a psychologist and a bone specialist. It's rather amusing looking back on the visits as, for some reason, I had it firmly fixed in my mind that the first doctor was the bone man. It sounds crazy, but it is an example of how you don't need to get much wrong to get it *all* wrong. For over an hour I answered all his questions as if he was a psychologist. With enormous difficulty I convinced myself that the question was based on psychology. I even commented to him that he appeared to understand a lot about bones. I was perplexed when he spent so long examining my chest X-rays. How was he trying to trick me? I took off my clothes as instructed and let him prod and feel my back and front. All this time warning bells were sounding in my head that things weren't 'quite right'.

It was not until I reached the next doctor for the afternoon who introduced himself as the psychologist that the penny dropped. This explained the ghastly trouble I experienced answering the last doctor's questions. I was so full of frustration that I didn't stop to ask for an explanation from the previous doctor. Just a few words would have thrown light on it all.

I was amazed at the number of times long and laborious eye tests had to be completed. It was most distressing, as somehow, the sight from my left eye was starting to be blocked out by my brain.

Doing Up Buttons

Another day, Ted drove me to a consultation with a psychiatrist who, in a very short time, decided I needed immediate hospitalisation and drugs for my depression. What I needed were explanations and empathy, not being locked away in a clinic. In my fragile state it was extremely difficult to walk out on an expert, a professional who had pre-judged what I needed. He even suggested I go straight from his rooms to the clinic, and that the family should bring in the things I needed after I had signed myself in. I suppose I was very lucky that Ted was waiting for me that day and I did not have to find a phone to get a cab.

The whole experience of travelling and waiting and trying to explain my difficulties to yet another stranger was very damaging to both body and soul.

By the time my civil action was to go to court my medical bills had reached over fifty thousand dollars. Apart from the physio, osteopath and my local GP, the initial hospital stay, neurologist, strabismus surgeons, neuropsychologist, cardiologist, orthopaedic surgeon and ophthalmologist my GP referred me to, the bulk of the money had been spent getting assessed. None of the assessments had made me any better, rather, if anything, the strain of travelling to the appointments had made me feel worse.

I'd never had anything to do with courts before, and had not realised that there are two different courts and their outcomes are based on different notions. In the criminal court, where the police had taken Mr X, things had to be proved beyond a reasonable doubt, whereas in the civil court, balance of probability is the main focus. If you are the person responsible for the accident, you cannot sue anyone. If only this were more generally known, I'm sure people would take greater care and be more responsible on our roads.

Helen tried to explain the court system to me, but at the time I was not capable of understanding or remembering the points. Only now can I understand and see the relevance of what she was saying. If I could have understood this at the time, I'm sure I would not have felt so sure I'd entered a crazy, mixed-up world. Helen has written up some notes to help me understand the system. These are included in the Help Section of the book.

Preparations for my civil case commenced a year after the accident. The case was eventually heard four years after the accident (apparently this is very fast for such an action). Helen wrote down the steps in a civil case for me. They were:

1 Make an appointment to see a solicitor – make sure it is a large firm that specialises in your area.
2 For the interview, bring along copies of all relevant documentation, and listen to the questions carefully. Answer any questions your solicitor may have and follow things up by letter. Remember to keep copies of everything you pass on to the solicitor, and try not to give him or her too many documents.
3 Procedures go before the court. Barristers are now involved.
4 Court. Firstly you are listed for court. The list may be called over. There may be too many cases timetabled for court, so your case is put off until another day.

Then comes your day in court. Australia has an adversarial system, which means having one side fight to disprove what the other side says.

To even get to the court steps was a mammoth task for me. First, there were the endless rounds of doctors. Take a person who is damaged, in pain a lot of the time, bewildered, afraid of venturing out in taxis, particularly to the city, and compel her to do a round of doctors and guess how she feels?

I found the build-up to the civil court case the most traumatic period of my life – I had eight different city doctors to visit in a few weeks. I saw three psychiatrists in one week, who all gave me the same IQ test. As a teacher, I knew that this test was invalid if taken more frequently than once a year! There was one psychiatrist who became very hostile and yelled at me, saying I was cheating because I could do parts of the test easily and had difficulty with the mathematical parts. I was beside myself with exhaustion: I was trying to hold down my part-time work and had to travel almost daily from far away and find out-of-the-way doctors' rooms for the medical appointments. Having a poor sense of direction and faulty memory made finding my way around the monolithic rabbit warrens of hospitals a nightmare. On more than one occasion I found myself sobbing in the gutter when trying to get a taxi home.

Words can't explain the trauma and frustration at being compelled to do what someone tells you. You are just powerless. I felt like screaming 'I don't want to be here! I just want to go home! Leave me alone!'

There were some kindly, helpful doctors on both my side and the other side. They could explain some of my difficulties,

In Court

which helped to fill in the jigsaw puzzle a little more.

One specialist, David de Horne, suggested that I visit the scene of the accident and place some flowers there. No-one had suggested doing such a thing to me before, but the idea really appealed. So, on the fourth anniversary of the accident, Ted and I returned to the scene. He stayed in the car while I ventured out in the rain with some gold ribbon and roses. I put my arms around that pole, near the blue paint from my car that was still there. I tied the ribbon around the pole, then tucked the bunch of roses into the ribbon and spoke to the pole and thanked it for not taking my life. I planted a soft kiss where my hard car had been smashed. When I got back into the car to join Ted, my cheeks were wet, not only from the rain. From that moment on, I felt something inside me start to heal.

The civil case was listed to take place on a Monday nearly four years after the accident. On the Friday before the case, I was made an offer, an out-of-court settlement. Apparently if I refused that offer, and lost the court case, I might be offered less money and be liable for the costs of going to court.

What should I do? Ted was interstate on business. I managed to locate him at an airport on his way home. Even though my diligent and helpful barrister was confident we would get more money if we went to court, I felt that a bird in the hand was worth two in the bush. I was afraid I might just die of fright in court. So on the Friday I decided to settle out of court.

I had said to Ted that I'd meet him in the city. But how could I thank my wonderful legal eagles? I had to do

Doing Up Buttons

something that afternoon so I walked down to the florist at the bottom of our hill who had made up and delivered so many beautiful bouquets to me. She made up two magnificent arrangements that I delivered, with grateful thanks, to my lawyers. I then met the family to celebrate with a very late afternoon tea.

When I got home I was beside myself with grief. Somehow, by accepting the offer, I felt as if I had sold out my situation, that I had made a trade with the devil. At dusk I slipped down into the garden and hugged the cool grey bark of a large lemon-scented gum, so like the telegraph pole, sobbing and begging, 'I'll give you back the money if you give me back my life!'

In the following weeks there was pleasure in giving some money to the kids so they could get something special, a reward for all they had done for me. I could spoil Ted too, and for myself I bought a warm winter's coat for standing in the street and waiting for taxis, and a beautiful ring. There was a lot of thought behind the purchase of this ring. It is something I have with me all the time. I had told myself then that the next time I felt like crying with frustration or self-pity I was to admire the ring instead. It was a celebration that I had a new start in life, a symbol that good can come from bad.

With the end of the court cases I thought that I would be free from appointments, that I would no longer have to see doctors if I didn't want to. But financial advisers have taken their place. Mr X still controls my life. I have tried to be careful and wise in investing the money as my future looks different with only part-time work. I only hope that I can make the settlement money subsidise my salary. Helen says that a large proportion of people who receive lump-sum payments go through their money in five years, no matter how large the sum is. I don't want to do that!

As Time Goes By

And in today already walks tomorrow.
— Samuel Taylor Coleridge

The summer came and went. We'd float on the swimming pool down the hill at the bottom of the garden, quietly watching ducks and water birds call to drink. On hot evenings we'd dine with the kids on the deck with candles flickering in the trees. As time passed it was possible to become more reflective about the accident and change.

Apart from visits to doctors, school, physio and my parents, all my time was spent at home. Ted or the children would take and assist me to shop for food. After two years I could walk for ten minutes down the hill to the milk-bar for milk. To carry even a litre of milk would mean that my shoulder and ribs would hurt the following day.

My friends have really been of great influence in helping me to cope. One afternoon, my dear friend Joyce took me out into Eltham for coffee. We'd shared many cups of coffee in the glass room but it took two years before she felt that going out would do me good. It was great to get out again. After we'd enjoyed our coffee and a chat, I decided that instead of troubling Joyce to drive me home I would go shopping on my own. I really needed a bra that would fit my misshapen winged figure. To complete the adventure, I would then walk home.

As Time Goes By

To be at the shops on my own was quite unique. I'd been wanting to shop for a bra for some time. The piece of shoulder bone sticking out pushed down any undergarment strap and my right 'wing' prevented any fitting properly. Finally, disappointed, desperate and embarrassed, I stumbled the two kilometres home with a bra that I hoped I could wear.

Writing helped me cope with such disappointments, frustration and sadness. I didn't want to burden the family with my whingeing; often I felt so self-indulgent already that I could not voice my moans to anyone any more. So I wrote them down. For example, on this day I recorded:

> The walk home from Eltham was interesting. Bare hawthorn hedges cascaded with birds silhouetted against the evening sky, yesterday's glory of colour now stark branches. The silence and solitude of the track, the little wooden bridge over the brown rushing waters of the creek trembles as I pass. I tap my way by peaceful fields of artichokes fringed with gum trees along the creek. Climbing up the hill now, and glimpses of the blue-mauve of the distant Dandenongs and Kinglake mountains against the pale lemon sky. Then down the steep slippery slope, along the fence beside the horse paddock. Lights are starting to twinkle in the valley. How often must my feet tread this path? How often must my stick tap-tap this track? How frequently must my gloved hand fumbled to touch a tree, a post, a branch searching for reality in this double world of mine? Oh Mr X, at the start of my walk home I cursed you, tears splashed down my face as car after car sped by me on the main road. I felt like an isolated outcast –

Doing Up Buttons

> everyone else could drive But to walk through the beauty of the valley made me aware how wonderful (and fragile) life is.

Another day I wrote:

> When trying on shoes today I had to ask the shop assistant to put the shoe on my left foot. No matter how hard I tried I just couldn't control my left leg. It felt as if someone had given me *their* left leg so of course I couldn't control it. This must be the same silly leg I don't know I've got when I have a shower, so I don't dry it afterwards. Then I try to push the wet thing out of bed. I wish I could get my own leg back again.

Some acquaintances would say, with just a touch of jealousy, 'What do you do with all the time on your hands?' I'm busy with doctors and physios and resting to get better, I reply. I thought of my unhappiness and frustration, and my passion to return to an active life like theirs. Change places with me, *please*! I couldn't tell of the silly little happenings that would drive me crazy as I was so dependent and constrained. So I wrote:

> Today I stood in a hardware shop as tears ran down my cheeks like the rain running down the window. Like the cloudburst outside, some dam burst in my head. Why was I crying? It was not that I had waited patiently thirty minutes for a taxi or waited patiently for another taxi just an hour before. Or that I'd waited patiently for the physio to use his magic hands to take away for a few hours the

As Time Goes By

pain I so patiently endured. It was the frustration of being powerless, of being trapped, of having no way out of this predicament. I could not change things by working or reasoning or creative thinking. All I could do was to find more patience. When the taxi eventually arrived, the driver was smoking and I had to ask him to put out the cigarette. Then I had to sit in the smelly, stuffy taxi for a frenetic, fast and furious trip home.

I had tried to set myself attainable goals. This time, I had felt really good. I'd really thought it through. I would walk from the physio's into the shops five minutes away. I would carefully cross the road to the hardware store to buy some glue for my cracked walking stick. I would cross the road again and buy a fresh iced bun for Ken and Rob to have for morning tea. Not much of a goal, but as I stood in the hardware shop with the storm outside I knew I couldn't walk across the road to get the bun to proudly present to my boys, to put a smile on their faces. Instead they had to mop up my face.

I think one of the most frustrating and upsetting things about the whole situation was the never-ending snowballing effects of having a damaged body. You never knew where the next ache or pain would come from. If you drag your leg, you get muscle spasm pains in the foot. Because you can't judge distance or heat levels, you constantly burn or hurt yourself – I would always be nursing a cut or burn or bruise. After two years I bent down one day and my lower rib twisted out, just like a powerful snake until it settled back. Would it poke right through my skin?

A visit to Hugh and Phillip my physio followed. I saw a bone surgeon who suggested that he remove the offending rib. I didn't want that. I've since discovered that if I extend one leg out in the air when bending down – rather like a ballet dancer – the build-up of force on my diaphragm that pops out my rib is released, and the rib stays where it is. Of course I sometimes forget that I need to act like a ballet dancer and it will pop out, catching me unawares.

I was in danger of becoming bitter and at times I still wonder whether life is worth living after having freedom and choice taken away. A great strain had been placed on Ted and the family. Rob, our younger son – the apple of my eye – was diagnosed with diabetes. Were the stresses and concern caused by my accident to blame for this?

The accident occurred at the time when my career had the most potential. As the weeks passed I became more and more aware of my difficulties, and the hope that I would return to my classroom slipped just a fraction from my grasp.

I find it so difficult not being free to drive. I know the chance of being in another accident is slight, but it has happened once. I have to steel myself to get in the car and I always ask 'Is this trip really worthwhile? Is it worth dying for?' Perhaps because the accident happened unseen from behind, I can never feel safe in a car again!

Social contact is difficult as I still have trouble understanding what people are saying. Somehow, music is no longer pleasurable and hurts my ears. Music that I have loved in the past somehow pulls directly on a chord that reminds me I'm not who I was.

Reading is no longer enjoyable; the theatre is difficult for

As Time Goes By

me to cope with; gardening, seeing, understanding and even walking is difficult with my balance and perception problems. Watercolour painting is difficult. Shopping and browsing are no longer a pleasure, because I tend to knock people and things over.

Dining out is difficult in noisy restaurants, even with ear plugs, so we have to eat out at 6 p.m. to avoid the crowds. I still spill food, or miss my mouth, or dribble down my chin.

I have had to give up my committee work with Life Education and Philosophy for Children. I am continuing teaching philosophy and extension work two mornings a week, and while this is a wonderful thing for now, what is to become of me in the future? I have had to learn to live with uncertainty.

At first I thought getting better would happen naturally, like day follows night. It has been the bitterest pill to swallow, to realise I will never be who I was. I don't know how much more improvement I can reasonably hope for. The accident has totally changed my capability to do the things that used to give me pleasure. It has also changed the amount of pleasure I get from doing those things I am still able to.

I am a very unlucky lucky person!

LIFE GOES ON

I've discovered that having a bad memory can be good – you can re-enjoy the same thing!
I've discovered that you can resent people who have power over you.

I suppose you could say I was buzzing around like a bee in a bottle, trying so hard to get better, to regain my lost life. I had an overwhelming determination to try and recapture as much of it as was humanly possible. I began to realise it would take longer than I had thought. In the past things had seemed straightforward, my goals attainable, shining on the horizon like the Emerald City in the Wizard of Oz. My road now had a big bend in it. The Emerald City could no longer be seen on the horizon; there were trees blocking any view of the horizon and my goals. Dangerous cliffs and rock slides on the road made every step forward a potential hazard. There were minefields all around me. At the same time, I was scanning everywhere for an opportunity, or something that might lead the way to some goal for the future.

I still had the wonderful hours I spent at school. The remainder of my time was spent resting. I scribbled poems on scraps of paper to try to capture what was happening to my life. These brief poems from the heart, along with the notes Helen and I prepared for the doctors and lawyers, helped me

Life Goes On

put together the first draft of this book. Once it had been accepted for publication I had a goal to work towards. This was empowering. To be happy, I needed to achieve something. Even capturing thoughts in an incomplete manner was an achievement – I was doing something.

I used many coping strategies during the course of these five years. It was sad as each anniversary passed and I wasn't 'better'. There was improvement, but in most cases, it was because I'd found ways of coping rather than the problem having improved dramatically. My energy was still being drained by my eyesight and the pain I was in.

I was driven, committed to trying to improve. I tried to focus on solving my numerous problems by trying to learn about and tackling different things that worried me. I realised that you don't get better, but that it's up to you to find ways to nibble away at the edges of problems until they are bearable. Just trying helps. I must confess that in the deep recesses of my mind I was still wishing for a miracle, that I'd wake up one morning and be able to see properly, that a new doctor would have a new way of helping, that my pain would melt away.

The eyepatch was driving me crazy. I asked my optician if there was such thing as a contact lens with an eyeball painted on it that would make me blind in the left eye. He did some investigating and found out about a business south of Brisbane that did such a thing. Ted and I travelled to the workshop, and discussed getting a lens to block out sight in my left eye. A couple of weeks later my third eye arrived. After I had got used to the contact lens I was feeling much less obvious out in public but a strange milkiness would cloud my vision when

Doing Up Buttons

I removed that eye. Investigation revealed that because of the paint on the lens my eye could not breathe and was being starved of oxygen. If I continued using the lens, I'd go blind in that eye. It might have been best at the time to have lost the use of my left eye, but I was having a lot of accidents because I got no warning of impending danger from it.

Helen rang me from work, very excited that a client also had a blocking-out third eye. I asked her to ask him about it on his next appointment. She rang me quite upset on the day of the appointment to tell me the sad news that he'd been run down and killed by a tram coming from his 'blind' side. My third eye went in the bin.

I then devised the idea of having dark tinted sunglasses for when I was out and about. Black paint covered the left lens, but I still had the peripheral warning vision out the side of the glasses, which helped me avoid walking into vehicles, walls and people.

Another disturbing facet of my faulty vision was that I could not identify an object if I was looking down at it. Also, I could not gauge steps and distance. An object, say, a tin of cat food, would be before me in the fridge but I would not be able to recognise it unless I bent down and had the object level with my face. To get a saucepan out of the cupboard required kneeling or lying on the floor so that my eye was level with the shelf. I could then see, but my knees then became the problem. Every gain I found seemed to have a corresponding loss, but I was learning to find ways to cope.

I suppose my swearing and ranting and raving and crying helped me reduce tension. At times I would just try to ignore

Life Goes On

the problems, but this would lead to pain the following day. Not wanting to be a nuisance to family and friends, I found myself withdrawing from the world. At other times I would try to concentrate on the positive or look for relaxing diversions.

Ted and I had some breaks away. As I hated being in a car, flights to Sydney or Canberra were pleasant diversions. Whenever the plane would tilt when taking off or landing I would feel panic, as I constantly feel like the ground is moving. I have found that looking at something close to my face helps block out the tilting other world. Overnight stays at Mount Macedon and Lorne were lovely. It was a bonus to be away from home and not have to walk to the shops or call for cabs or have to deal with doctors or physios. It was a real break from routine.

The family had their own ways of coping. Rob now says the effect of the accident on him was like a whip that made him recoil. He socially withdrew, stunned and confused. He didn't ask the common question 'Why has this happened?' Instead, he seemed to accept it on one level and gradually sorted out the issues over a long period of time. Ann was busy running the house; she was doing so much to help, being both cook and bottle-washer, nurse and cheerleader. Ken and Helen had their uni life and studies to escape to, and Ted's time was taken up with a very hectic workload at the office, and a stoic belief that we just had to hang in there. He relieved stress by doing things to help me when he got home.

The Good Times Start to Come Again

I've discovered that you need to like what you do, not do what you like, to be happy.

After two years we realised that recovery was going to take longer than we'd all thought. Predictably that had its ups and downs. I fell down, I got up, put a band-aid on my knees, and struggled on till my next fall.

My fiftieth birthday turned out to be a time of being up. Birthday celebrations at home are always doubled in pleasure as Ted's birthday is the day following mine. The Friday of my birthday dawned wet, chilly and miserable – fairly much in tune with how I felt – 'down' and aching. I'd been wrestling with one of my nasty and numerous chest infections for a couple of weeks.

As a treat, the whole family was to spend the night at Queenscliff. After an Aspro Clear cocktail that afternoon, Ken drove me to the city where Ted picked me up for our big adventure. Off we went, full of optimism. We arrived at our destination in a flurry of squalls and dashed from the dreadful weather to the warm, welcoming, lit and orderly Queenscliff Hotel. Bliss.

Orchids from my friend Helen were in our room. There was a joyous festive feeling as the family gradually took over the first floor, safely in from the cold.

Ted produced an exquisite ring – what a surprise and a thrill! We gathered in front of a roaring fire in the front parlour while the whole family sat round in their glad rags. I felt like a queen going into the beautiful candle-lit dining-room surrounded by the jewels of our family.

After dinner we sat in the charming sitting-room where the kids played chess and card games. Outside the storm raged. Inside we were cosy and cheery. We had weathered the storm.

Helen and Greg's wedding was celebrated at Montsalvat in Eltham the following year. The early morning sun glowed through the beautiful old windows as they stood barefoot and crowned with wheat – a joyous happening.

Ann and Tony were wed a year later at dusk, also at Montsalvat. The dark pool was twinkling with dozens of floating candles and strains of jazz played through the starlit velvet sky.

Marcus and Deb were wed in a quaint cliff-top chapel on Phillip Island a month later.

Mum and Dad were there for all the weddings. The family was together. Wonderful.

Examining the Heart

Ignorance is never better than knowledge.
　　　　　– Enrico Fermi

It was a sunny afternoon. Ted and I were wandering in Carlton and we decided to browse in Readings, the local bookshop. Ted was engrossed discovering interesting books and I decided I'd try to select a book to read. I'd read only a handful of books in the past few years. Maybe I could rediscover the bookworm side of me? But what book could I choose? Not one about travel – if you can't travel you're no longer interested in the subject. I searched through the other books – there were no paperbacks with print large enough for me to read, or with reasonable spaces between the lines. I didn't want crime or anything frightening. Nothing sad either.

Suddenly it hit me. Just like Jenny, the mother of one of my pupils who was very ill with cancer, I've lost my interest to read. If things are too shallow they're not worthwhile, otherwise they are too scary. This was a sad revelation. This discovery brought to the surface the sadness and frustration that were bubbling, almost out of control, beneath the exterior of my life.

The experience of facing the reality of things lost led me to confide in Hugh, my dear GP. After some discussion he referred me to a psychologist. He said she was a delightful lady and that we should get on well together.

My first visit to June left me seething. How dare this person tell me I didn't know who I was before the accident! How dare she suggest I was experiencing difficulties! I tried frantically to sweep my sadness under the mat and deny that I was lost and depressed. 'I'll never come back, so there!' I kept telling myself as I sat through our first session.

My homework was to write down things that gave me some pleasure. Now, this got me in and stirred my curiosity. I didn't think that I got much pleasure from anything any more. Almost against my will, I secretly noted down things as they came to mind. My list included achieving something, Ted and the kids being home, nature, having a hot shower for the pain, tapestry, drinking coffee in the sun, feeding the birds and having Steff, our dog, by my side. Wow! This was powerful stuff. Even if things were fairly insignificant, there was some pleasure in my pain.

For the next visit I took my list and a diary I was keeping to share with June. I explained that I could not remember my way around my own house; I couldn't find the tap to turn off the hose; I keep expecting Rob to be ten, not seventeen; I felt trapped, disempowered and dependent; my career was gone; I was pushy with the family; I felt I didn't belong at school; I was angry and frustrated, and felt as if I was just going through the motions of life. Everyone, including me, expected me to be better by this time, but I wasn't. I felt I was constantly disappointing everyone. June explained that we would work slowly through the issues, and try to find a level where I felt comfortable.

Doing Up Buttons

June discovered that I had three main issues to resolve. First, I had to stop pretending that I was happy when I wasn't, that I understood people when I didn't. Secondly I did not want to be constantly disappointed in myself. Thirdly I did not want to be consistently frustrated. Also, I wondered if there was an alternative to having to pay for everything I did in pain and exhaustion.

This was June's summary of my situation:

> There were signs that Christine's struggle to recapture her old self was taking too much of a toll. Problems were developing around her trying to redefine herself to some extent, rather than try to retrieve her old self. Christine found this notion terrifying at first, most probably because she has been hanging on to her identity and roles like grim death in the face of great physical and some mental changes. (The mental changes in automatic functions such as memory, retrieving words, the concept of number etc, rather than in her cognitive functioning per se, which seems intact. However, these changes in automatic mental functions have been devastating in routine areas of life.)
>
> This hurdle of allowing for such changes in a new persona was causing her some difficulty and protracting her grief. Much of her emotional energy was going into a battle to become more like she was in the past, rather than exploring the important issue of what she could enjoy and thrive on now. She is doing extremely well in creating more flexibility in her outlook and pursuits, and has shown very good insight and capacity for adaptation and change. As Christine progressed it became apparent

that her family was to some extent stuck in the same way she had been, and were unsure of how to respond to her problems.

Christine has endeavoured to fight off major changes in physical and mental ability. She has persisted too long in the attempt to retrieve the person she was, at the expense of recognising the pain she was experiencing and exploring alternative paths of growth and development. She appears to have numerous skills, and over time will be likely to develop associated or new areas of expertise and enjoyment. She may also retain older areas of skill, and moderate or otherwise alter her involvement in them or her approach to them. As Christine has begun to accept herself as she is now rather than trying to push herself back into her previous mould, her peace of mind is returning and her grief resolving.

June suggested all sorts of solutions to cope with my problems. For example, to go late to the cinemas to avoid the road trauma ads. I've since decided that the best thing is to ask at the ticket office – they can tell you if they are screening the ads. (I went to the movies with a friend and when an ad came on the screen she said she couldn't see my heels for dust. One minute I was sitting beside her, the next I was gone. I think she found me sobbing in the lobby!)

Another suggestion of June's was that I should always sit in an aisle seat when in public places. June explained that there was no actual danger in places such as a store, the danger was in my mind. This certainly helped with the panic attacks when I feel trapped by people. We had goals of pushing back my threshold of panic to assist in desensitising myself. June also explained that I can't do anything when in the middle of an attack, that I just had to wait for the adrenalin to go.

I also had to learn to be content with nibbling around the edges of my trauma. Knocking off little bits at a time helped to lighten the weight, and I slowly learnt to cope by breaking up big tasks into small, more manageable, things. This reminds me of a story I used to tell my new students at the beginning of the new school year. It was story of the 'Strong Man' show in a nearby Civic Centre. The strongest man in the world pulled and pulled at a phone book, trying to tear it apart with his bare hands. He inquired if there was any one in the audience who could do this. A little girl in the back row put up her hand. In disbelief the Strong Man invited her on stage to demonstrate. With every eye on her the lass walked up the aisle, up the stairs and on to the stage. She calmly took the large phone book and purposefully set about tearing each page in two.

I learnt to go into a shop and ask for bread or bananas without crying. I slowly found my way to and from doctors' appointments in the city without panicking.

One sunny morning June made the most unbelievably helpful suggestion. She said, 'Chris, what would you say if I said a friend from work had head injuries and was experiencing all the problems you have outlined to me?' Of course I said how sorry I'd feel for them, how I'd tell them to slow down, that their mistakes don't matter. June then said something quite startling. She said I had to learn to treat this damaged side of myself – the one I called my bumbling idiot – as if she was my own best friend! So instead of being hostile and critical of this other me, I had to try to be kind

Examining the Heart

and helpful. I would say to my best friend – in my head – 'Don't worry, let's write that down so you don't forget it, let's make a list.'

It was wonderful to have June to tell my secrets to. I still thought I was mad or at least very thick. One day I looked out the window and although it wasn't raining I could see water falling on one part of the drive. Wow! This is weird! This is exciting. I returned to the window to look at the drive several times over the next half-hour or so. What was happening? Should I ring the newspaper to get someone to witness this incredible phenomena? I then forgot the whole episode and later when I went to get the letters I saw that the hose was on. It took me a few minutes to realise that *this* was the magic rain from heaven!

Another day I saw circles on the gravel drive. A similar flood of wonderment and trying to make sense of the occurrence happened in my head – visitors from outer space? The same creatures who made the circles in the crops in England?

As I was leaving the school-ground one day I saw a mother talking to a tree. 'Oh the poor thing! I wonder if she is all right? Now what should I do? Take her to the principal? Go and make her a cup of coffee? How can I help?' After what seemed a long time exploring possibilities, her friend, who was standing behind the tree moved into view ...

June said I was to stop the creative side of my brain from taking over. If anything seemed weird or odd I had to check all the information available and go back to something I understood. I had to look at *facts* and widen my knowledge base before I could come to a conclusion.

Doing Up Buttons

In retrospect, I believe these were all indications of my incredible one-track mind. It was so hard to understand or form thoughts. Any distraction would mean I entirely lost what I was saying or thinking. My way of coping was to hang on to an idea like grim death!

So gradually my best friend and I learnt to enjoy things. Progress was measured according to what I had achieved in a week or a month. According to June, I seemed to have only two speeds – flat out fast and stationary. Looking after my best friend let me try the steady-as-she-goes routine (well, when I remembered).

Disorientation in the morning still troubled me greatly. I would wake up not knowing who I was and what day it was. Somehow this was a strange, private proof that this bumbling idiot had taken over my body. It has taken me five years to be able to wake up and say, 'Today is Thursday. On Thursdays I ...' Ted found it strange when I lay in bed some mornings looking upset and puzzled just because I didn't know what day it was. 'There's nothing to worry about – I'll *tell* you what day it is each day,' he assured me. That was not the point, but like so many problems, the solution was a simple one – a page-by-page calendar by my bed that I could turn over every morning to see the day and schedule.

Taxis were another trauma on my list. June helped me to see that I'd go out for a spot of shopping and then push myself so hard while I was out and about that before I knew it, I'd be over my threshold of tiredness. This explained why I had spent miserable times sitting in the gutter, sobbing as if my heart was broken, all because I couldn't get a taxi! June suggested that I should always have a plan for where I'll get a taxi from. When I'm in the city I can go to a taxi rank at any of the large hotels. If no taxi comes to the rank, I should go and have a coffee somewhere, have a rest, *then* try again. Even though it felt like the end of the world and all I wanted was *bed*, it wasn't the end of the world.

I also carried a list in my bag entitled 'What to do when I don't know what to do'. Suggestions included sit down, don't panic, have a coffee, ring Ted or Ken. I've tried booking a taxi before I leave home to pick me up at the other end, but without fail, something would come up or I'd bump into someone who could give me a lift or I'd be running late. Having a phone card or the right coins for the phone is such an obvious thing, but I actually needed June to point out the obvious. Last birthday both Ted and Marcus had the same surprise for me – yes, you've guessed it, a mobile phone!

I believed June when she explained that school was taking up all my effort, but I still hung on like grim death.

Facing the Music

Take away love and our earth is a tomb.
　　　　　—Robert Browning
(Wo)Man — A being in search of meaning.
　　　　　—Plato

We used to have a darling brown poodle called Beaver Brown. On the day we bought him we took him to the beach, where he delighted the children with his antics: trying to drink the seawater, falling cutely in the depressions in the sand and displaying curiosity in everything. That night, as we were tucking Beaver Brown up with his hot-water bottle and clock, we saw he was having trouble breathing.

'Oh no,' we thought, 'we've been sold a pup! He's sick! Curses!'

So we made an after-hours visit to the vet. To our astonishment, the vet took a pair of tweezers and started to pull out a tiny splinter, no thicker than a hair, that he'd noticed in the pup's neck. He pulled and pulled, and to our shock, out came a three-inch grass seed. It was just like watching a magician doing a trick, as we gaped at this long grass seed that had worked itself into Beaver's flesh. How thankful we were that we'd taken the dog to the vet that evening. By morning his throat may have been so swollen he could have choked. That grass seed was invisible, unimagined, yet so dangerous!

Facing the Music

June found the tiny tip of an idea-seed poking out of me. It took many months with June before this secret seed that was growing so deep beneath the surface could poke a tentative shoot to the light of day. It was an example of how what you believe influences what you see.

Ted had been *wonderful*, Ted had done so much for me, Ted had made his life revolve round me. But I felt guilty, ashamed and disgusted in myself. I felt so pathetic, hopeless and helpless, I believed *no-one* could love me. I knew I was not the girl he had married so long ago, nor was I the same woman he was married to before the accident. So I searched for proof that he didn't love me!

Daily there was evidence of his care for me, but I was blind to that. Instead, I was fixated on looking for proof that he didn't care. I became totally absorbed in the idea that, 'If he loved me he would have done what I wanted.' If he loved me he would have sat beside me, he wouldn't have let me be tortured by the physio or left me in the hospital in the multi-bed ward. How could he poke an eight-minute microwaved egg into me and consider that helping? June suggested that I should talk about these notions that were stifling me. So I tentatively mentioned it to the kids. They said in astonishment, 'Mum, Dad was with you the whole time you were in Intensive Care . . . he hardly came home.' But I was unconscious at the time . . . I didn't know that he'd been with me! Oh dear!

Once I was out of danger – and conscious – Ted would pop in to see me on his way to and from work. I would lie there, thinking, 'His job is more important/has higher priority than me', when he was just trying to hold on to his job, and make up for some of the time he had spent with unconscious me! He was also so shocked by all that had happened that he just wanted to escape from the hospital once he knew I was going to survive!

As for having me shifted to another hospital, it hadn't entered his head – he thought I was receiving the best care where I was. He was having trouble coping. He was a man of action. When he fed me the egg he was doing something to help.

I needed empathy, Ted needed to fix things. June gently showed me that it was lack of understanding, *not* lack of love, on Ted's part.

Once this grass seed was extracted, and I could examine it in the light of day, the painful swelling could subside and I could breathe, think and live anew.

What I believed had influenced how I perceived things. Confusingly, at other times, the reverse was true: I could only believe in something once I had seen it, or someone else had seen it!

My appointment with Dr Maureen Malloy was a mind-opener. I had been sent to so many specialists. I never knew if they would have any effect on my pain, sight or understanding. This time I got the door prize – a wise, empathetic and understanding doctor. She treated me like a person, not a patient. She could understand my difficulties.

I had spent so many specialist visits trying to explain all my problems. Until I saw Dr Malloy, no specialist had appeared to understand. No-one had explained that the symptoms I was experiencing were typical of head injury. I was starting

Facing the Music

to believe that I must be mad, or just imagining things that were not real.

Dr Malloy was an example that seeing proof, or evidence, affects what we believe. After giving me a test she would look at the results. She would then translate the results into something I could understand. Dr Malloy would suggest, for example, that perhaps I had difficulty following conversations in the school staff room. Good heavens, this was true! I knew I felt uncomfortable in a group, that I found it hard, but I had not analysed why! My faulty short-term memory was why I couldn't follow conversations!

Like a magician pulling rabbits out of a hat she could explain some of the unseen and unspoken things that were in my 'hat'. Here was someone to show me my problems, instead of me trying to express my shortfalls. Now I could really believe they existed!

The relief was profound. For several years I'd felt guilty for not trying harder to make things 'right', for sweeping many uncomfortable events under the carpet. I'd felt so bad that I was not looking at the positive things in life: of how lucky I was to be alive, that I didn't have worse injuries, as had been suggested to me. Now I knew my problems were real!

This perceptive doctor explained that my thoughts flow too quickly for my memory. She gave me strategies for coping with this strange world I found myself in.

1 Touching things to help me focus.
2 If I was trying to remember something, to shut my eyes to visualise without distractions.
3 As I could only cope with small amounts of information,

to break information into manageable chunks. This was so helpful: from thinking only of the spoons when setting the table to breaking telephone numbers into two or three digits at a time.
4 I needed *time* to get a meaningful idea in my mind.
5 I needed to set priorities:
- To learn to be comfortable with myself.
- To zipper my mouth so that I was not annoying my family by asking them to repeat things and endlessly explain.
- To keep my thoughts to myself.
- To remember that it *doesn't matter* if I miss out on some things – I do not need to be always struggling and fretting, trying to understand.
- To be a willow and bend with life's forces, and not try to remain rigid and unyielding.

Mum and Dad

Their love was boundless, their adventurous spirit unquenchable, their sense of fun legendary, and their creativity and wisdom only exceeded by their universal generosity.
  – Plaque on my parents' memorial rose bush

My parents were a constant source of support, and hardly a day passed without some contact with them. For the first couple of years after the accident they would make the long journey from Black Rock to Eltham regularly and sit with us by the fire in winter, or on the deck in summer, to try to encourage us. I feel so sorry that for the last four years of their lives my condition was a constant concern to them. Our visits home for coffee and a chat around the round table in the sun-room were a comfort. There is nothing like returning to the home of your childhood, being spoilt by your parents, and wandering in the garden.

Our visits were always an occasion for them. The smell of brewing coffee would greet us at the front door, ahead of Dad, with his arms wide open for a bear hug. There would always be something special, like freshly baked cream kisses or a piece of bitey cheese. Everything would be in readiness and it felt so good to be the highlight of their day. Even though they were elderly it seemed OK for them to fuss and look after and spoil me. We'd leave with flowers from the garden and something as a treat for the family.

Ted's parents had been neighbours and close friends of my parents for over fifty years. Ted's dad had died some years ago. His mum's health was not good and she had to be moved into a nursing home. Her life had been devoted to music. She had been my music teacher and confidant during Mum and Dad's regular overseas visits. I'd had lessons at their home across the road. I can remember my hands sticking to the piano keys during lessons when Ted, on returning from school, would pop his head round the door to ask what there was to eat. He's not the boy next door but the boy across the road!

The fourth year after my accident, Ted's Mum died, and my mother's health was deteriorating to such an extent that Dad could no longer care for her at home. The week she was installed in a nursing home near their home, Dad was diagnosed with leukemia. Sadness and guilt haunt me because I was of so little support to them during their final months. I would make the hour-long journey by taxi once a week to try to spend some time with Dad, then Ted, who worked nearby, would take us to visit Mum.

Dad mastered the computer and wrote a wonderful book about his life. I am so ashamed that I did not read his manuscript when he gave it to me. Reading was so difficult but I should have asked Ted to read it to me so that Dad and I could discuss it during the pleasant afternoons we shared together. We had wonderful philosophical discussions about life. He enjoyed telling me stories of his childhood. Some of his stories helped to cancel out the bad feelings I had.

By a strange quirk of fate, Dad's favourite spot when he

Mum and Dad

was a lad living in Kew was by the Yarra River, only a few metres from where my accident occurred. I thought of the spot with horror until Dad spoke of the thrill he'd had as a boy, of seeing a beautiful row of Canadian canoes and rowing skiffs, full of inviting colourful cushions for hire. As you floated down the river on a Sunday afternoon, he said, you knew you were getting close to the boathouse as the sound of the gramophone came into earshot. Dad's ghosts of memories changed my ghastly memories of the spot.

Dad frequently spoke about his 'guardian angel'. My ears always pricked up to Dad's stories of his 'guardian angel'. (I had one myself – a flesh-and-blood one – Peter!) At times in Dad's life his angel must have worked overtime. When he was about four and was on holiday with his family at Belgrave, he found his father's Harrington & Richards shotgun in the wardrobe. Dad could hardly lift the gun, let alone hold it to his shoulder.

'None the less I was playing with it, making all the appropriate noises. My grandmother was in the living room reading when I pointed it towards her and said "Bang Bang."

'She said, "Dear, take it away, I hate guns." So I took it into the passage just six feet away. Pointing it towards the back door I pulled the trigger and said bang again. There was a terrific explosion; the recoil sent me hurtling backwards. The back door had completely vanished.'

Dad was always keen to discuss my lessons and add suggestions, and before long, school-day and teacher stories would follow. His earliest school days were sweetened by the words of encouragement Miss Grey, his teacher, said when she'd praised his plasticine 'sparrow'. He had the pleasure of helping her with a hearing aid when she was an old lady, and discovered

Doing Up Buttons

that she regarded encouragement as the greatest gift a teacher could have.

Encouragement was at the heart of another of Dad's stories. On a cold grey day (when I was a year old) Dad was wandering around the grounds of the US institution made famous by Helen Keller, when he was invited to observe a young lady teaching a sweet little girl who was deaf and blind. When he was leaving, he tried to express some of his emotion and admiration. To his surprise the teacher burst into tears. She was on the point of giving up. She spoke of discouragement and the slowness of results, but Dad's visit had renewed her spirit. The weather was even more dismal when he left the building but he felt he was walking on air.

'Chick, we can never know the importance of words of encouragement,' he would say.

Dad once met and spoke to Helen Keller. He would recount her famous words about how sometimes we look at the door 'that's just closed in our faces so long, we fail to see the door opening just up the road a little'.

I would tell him of my frustration of being unable to find out about my condition, how specialists would treat me as a 'case', a 'statistic', and not a person.

We'd reminisce about the past; Dad, I'm sure, doing it to encourage me, and ensure that I never lost hope. There was the time his grandfather had said, 'Markie, we are all just like ants on a summer's day.' Dad, at the tender age of five, had no idea of what the words meant (expressing the brevity of man's existence and his insignificance in a boundless universe) but the way his grandfather treated him like a 'person' left a lasting memory.

Mum and Dad

He spoke of returning home to Black Rock in the summer evenings during their early days of marriage to find Mum on the heath-fields picking flowers in the moonlight. When Marcus and I were growing up we had a bathing box and a little boat moored nearby. Summer evenings would be heavenly.

Mum and Dad loved practical jokes. I well remember the one that backfired. Each afternoon, when I was about ten, I'd return from school and Mum would hide herself in the house somewhere for me to find. One afternoon I eventually located her squashed into the narrow broom cupboard. We had to wait for Dad to get home from work to dismantle the cupboard to release her!

Mum had been in the nursing home for only three months when she fell and broke her hip. She developed pneumonia when she was recovering.

One day Dad made the Christmas cake and pudding and visited Mum, who was most unwell, several times during the day. The next day he was desperately ill with an infection. Mum died several days later, during an afternoon when I was with her. Dad, who was in hospital receiving transfusions, passed away three days later.

At the funeral Mum and Dad were united in one coffin. We had baskets of oranges for guests to take home as a memento of how they met – Mum's bag of oranges broke and Dad had picked them up for her.

Their rose bush is just across a path from Ted's parents' grave. They are still neighbours.

The Encouragement Process

Words are, of course, the most powerful drug used by mankind.
— Rudyard Kipling

Dad was constantly speaking about people's great need to have appreciation, approbation and encouragement. Encouragement has been a strong thread, like gold, woven through my life. It has helped me to cope. I was fortunate that my part-time work at school gave me the opportunity to attend conferences about enrichment.

At one conference I was held spellbound by an entertaining and fascinating speaker, Dr Felice Kauffmann. Felice was speaking about underachievement among gifted students. As she spoke it was if the sky parted, allowing a sunbeam to illuminate a great truth. All she had to say about the underachieving student was so relevant to me, an adult who had experienced a loss of identity. Felice said that characteristics of the discouraged person include lack of confidence, thoughts of worthlessness, avoidance of responsibility, avoidance of competition, need for power and control, and close-mindedness.

Imagine being forced to engage in a task that you find utterly terrifying or repugnant. It might be an ordinary task, such as filling out forms, losing weight, speaking in front of a large group, or one that requires great heroics, such as

The Encouragement Process

performing brain surgery or engaging in combat. Now suppose that while you are reading this, someone locks you in a room and forces you to perform the task over and over again. Imagine that you remain locked in that room for an entire week . . . or a month. Finally, imagine that your 'sentence' has been extended and you will be locked in the room to perform the task every day for the rest of your life.

I suddenly understood that it takes real courage to tackle the problems experienced by someone who has had an accident. It is a life sentence. They certainly need encouragement – 'The giving of courage'.

My dictionary defines encouragement as 'To make bold, to put heart into, to urge, to promote courage'. How do we do this? Kindness, interest, sympathy, empathy, an ear to listen and a warm smile can all encourage you to press on. This is another instance where something small can have a big effect. A friendly cheery word from doctors' receptionists, taxi-drivers or shopkeepers can keep you going all day. Like Dad said, a little encouragement can go a long way! Genuine praise is also encouraging. Knowledge empowers and revitalises. When we know about something we can try to understand, accept and progress.

It's difficult to define encouragement tangibly, so perhaps it's easier to think of some of the things that discourage. These include domination, insensitivity, silence and intimidation. Powerlessness and the domination of others over me, by everyone from the specialists to my own family, were scary. Even though all of this was for my own good, the attitude crushed me. At the same time, the pressure to do the right thing was driving me nuts. Being in this heightened state of

Doing Up Buttons

sensitivity and having to bear the brunt of other people's insensitivity – who perhaps just wanted to say something positive, and would remark how wonderful I looked and how great my progress was – seemed insincere. Especially when I had just stumbled or spilt my dinner down my front. How hard it is for onlookers to compliment or praise a person who experiences such difficulty in everything that they do!

On the other hand, silence can be devastating when you have achieved something that might in itself be small, but for you, a huge leap forward. I am very fortunate that my family noted and expressed pleasure at each and every faltering step, but I would imagine it was a constant commitment and was fraught with danger! As a past perfectionist, I was always judging my self-worth by my accomplishments. I was programmed to be a human do-er, not a human be-ing. I felt totally worthless, discouraged and without hope because my hands and mind were frozen, and I was not capable of doing what I wanted to.

THE YEAR OF THE DOVE

There is nothing either good or bad but thinking makes it so.
— Shakespeare
I've discovered that mind power is amazing . . .
I've discovered what doesn't kill you makes you stronger.

Today it's five years since that day my life changed. I woke up feeling very sad. As the day progressed I pondered why this was so. Every other year this had been a time of family celebration of life and survival.

Why did I feel so bad this year? Then I realised why. I still hurt most of the time and I still couldn't see. I'd been telling myself, 'Be patient and you'll be better in the future!' My idea of the future was obviously five years.

I was wallowing in self-pity and couldn't get my act together. At school a dear little lass sat down beside me and declared out of the blue, 'I love you'. During the workshops the kids analysed and argued and laughed. I'd pushed myself but, yes, it was worth it. I was recording some of the 'Pearls of Wisdom' the students had shared – some of their secrets of life – and suddenly I thought, 'Pull up your socks – the kids have a lot of wisdom and encouragement for life, listen to them.'

So, on reflection, I've come a long way. I've learnt so much. I can stumble, fall, and get lost without feeling bad. I realise that I get exhausted, so most of the time I take things gently and I get by with a nap on most days. The days I don't have a nap I may need to take a sleeping pill at night because I'm over-tired but that's OK too. When I'm out, I sit for a coffee when I'm exhausted, and the mobile phone makes me feel I have some control over getting taxis or being able to contact someone. I have a wire trolley to help me carry milk and bread up the hill.

Physically I still experience a fair degree of pain in my shoulder and ribs (both front and back). A weekly visit to Jeremy, my wonderful osteopath, seems to pop my ribs back in and keeps the pain bearable. I often have the sensation that I've a tomahawk embedded in my back, but I can cope. I have to always take care when bending or doing up shoelaces so that my lower ribs do not pop out.

The double vision at times drives me crackers. I've tried corrective lenses and they only make matters difficult in a different way. Thank goodness I have not had my eyes operated on. It may have been like the glasses, only permanent. My balance has improved somewhat, but when I least expect it, I stumble. I've realised that when I turn around is when I'm at most risk.

I have a much closer relationship with Ted. After the initial trauma – as Ted puts it – 'With all the best will in the world it requires a great degree of acrobatic expertise to make love to a woman with a smashed skeletal frame' – we have proved that with time, gentleness and love, all things are possible.

It is only now that I am starting to realise what he has gone through. I don't expect him to be a mind-reader, although frequently he can guess what I am trying to say with only a

The Year of the Dove

few strange clues. I can now ask for what I want or need. Ted has been a tower of strength to lean on and also the wind beneath my wings. Love has pushed and pulled me to recover to the degree I have. Ted and the family's encouragement, patience, innovation and love have not only changed the world for me, but changed me for the world. I am so thankful.

The other morning Ted and I stood on the deck, spellbound at the visit of a pair of exquisite king parrots. These superb creatures were quite unconcerned as they breakfasted from the bird feeding-tray not far from where we stood. Their colours were vivid. As it was a foggy morning they shone like two bright jewels floating in milk. Birds have been a happy thread running through my days.

Ted spoke of the importance of the accident in his life in that it has helped him prioritise issues, and showed that relationships are more precious than anything else. He is constantly reminded that situations are not static.

Five years ago, in my first agonising days at home, Ken had tried to interest me in a couple of tame white doves that had been pensioned off by a magician. This absolutely captivated my imagination – oh, to have a 'Bird of Peace', a 'Bird of Hope', a 'magic bird' to sit on your shoulder! (Not the parrot I felt I needed to complete the effect when I wore the eyepatch.) But there were no more doves to be had. The kids then decided that they would get me some ordinary doves.

For weeks they became architects and designed countless quaint, weird and amazing dove-cotes. Time passed. The pile of design drawings grew, pages torn or photocopied from books and magazines joined the pile. This labour of love became a point of contention as no-one could decide the winning design for the Dove Taj Mahal. The whole idea was dropped. Secretly I was a little disappointed. I didn't really mind what the dove-cote was like, I really fancied some doves!

On the day of the fifth anniversary of the accident Ken rang me so see if I was OK. He sounded very pleased with himself. Apparently there was a month-old fan-tail dove at Montsalvat that was being pecked by the other birds in the aviary. Would I like it?

I jumped at the chance! That evening Ken arrived home with a bedraggled, pathetic grubby white bundle of feathers in a cardboard box. It had no tail feathers yet, and because of the way it pushed up its chest when it tried to stand it had no balance. Oh, so like a white ghost of me five years ago.

It was love at first sight, and the little dove nestled up to me, sitting contentedly on a towel on my knee. When Helen saw us together she christened it 'Lovey-dovey'.

Lovey's tail is now a beautiful snowy fan. Her mother, 'Cloud', has also come to live with us. She's a beautiful white bird, but she's timid and doesn't appear to enjoy human company like Lovey. Lovey now spends much of her day with me, sitting on my shoulder snuggling into my hair and neck while I work on the computer. We have 'flying lessons' where she takes off and usually returns to perch on my arm or Steff's head. My days are full of the music of the cooing of the doves.

At first I was really concerned because the fan-tails seemed so ridiculous: they were not able to fly without flapping, were awkward both on the ground and in the air. I would say to them, 'Oh you poor different things – what use are you –

you're not an animal and not a true flying bird, you poor little things.' And then I found out why they were bred like that. Their purpose is to fly and flap in the air, causing a commotion for the homing pigeons to see, to be a beacon in the air above their home so that the other normal pigeons can return safely.

Again, so much like me! Awkward, different, not seeing like normal people. Perhaps this book is like the furious fluttering of wings and tail to point the way, to mark the spot so that people, not pigeons, can find some peace, a resting place of the mind after their long journey from another place.

POSTSCRIPT:
THE WILD GOOSE CHASE

What lies behind us and what lies before us are tiny matters compared with what lies within us.

– In the office of Brooklyn Heights School (USA)

I now believe that victims of trauma have to gather and process as much varied, helpful information as possible to help them understand their condition. With determination, courage, hope and damn hard work, life can show some improvement. But still my mind was full of wondering. Is this the whole story? Where can I find out more about head injuries and the experiences of others? What is the secret of success? These questions were to eventually lead us on a wild goose chase to find the golden egg of advice.

Helen won a Queen's Scholarship to assist her study for a doctorate in law at New York University. Like the weird and wonderful plants that were starting to pop up in the garden where Lovey and Cloud had spilt their pigeon-food mix, three shoots slowly emerged in the dark recesses of my mind.

First, I wanted to go to New York to visit and support Helen. Secondly, maybe in the US I could find out more about head injury as the greater population meant there would be a greater number of brain injury (BI) sufferers. Thirdly, there was also a tiny shoot of hope that maybe someone

Postscript: The Wild Goose Chase

would be able to do something about my eyes.

And so Ted and I set off. Helen greeted us at the airport and took us to her apartment at Brooklyn Heights. She had worked like a beaver to tee up contacts in rehab and doctors for me to see. Appointments were made. On the week that we had no appointments, the three of us travelled to Boston to see the autumn leaves and Cape Cod. We had great difficulty getting accommodation as it was a holiday weekend. After numerous phone calls we obtained lodgings at the John Jeffries House. From the dark and drizzle of the evening we entered an ordered and lovely old rest-house. We got to our rooms and I pushed back the curtains to look out into the night. The first thing I saw was a large sign on the building across the street: Massachusetts Eye and Ear Infirmary.

Maybe someone here could help me! On reading the literature of our hotel it became apparent that this was used to house people visiting the Infirmary. Curiouser and curiouser, as Alice would say! After many phone calls – and more than a little pushing – I obtained an appointment to consult a Dr Natalie Azar at 9 the following morning.

The doctor was a delight: she talked about when she'd spent some time in Sydney as a teenager. After a lengthy consultation, where she explained to Ted how I was seeing. Double vision was her field of expertise. She felt confident that surgery could help me. She also said that she understood the complexities and that only a small number of doctors were *au fait* with my situation. She said there was one doctor in Australia whom she was certain could help me. His practice was just a half-hour drive from my home. I don't need to describe our delight or amazement.

Doing Up Buttons

When we returned to Helen's quaint apartment we made numerous calls to anyone we could trace to do with BI.

Someone told us of a head injury (HI) meeting and Ted and I attended the first meeting of the Brooklyn Chapter of the HI Association. Here, we were presented with some American statistics:

- Every 15 seconds someone in the United States will suffer a brain injury.
- An estimated 500 000 to 700 000 people in the US require hospitalisation each year from brain injuries, and an estimated 100 000 people die as a result of their injury.
- The average age of BI survivors is 15–25 years of age. Half of all BI survivors are under the age of 35.

After hearing Dr John Ryder speak for twenty minutes I whispered in Ted's ear, 'It was worth the trip just for these past twenty minutes!'

The doctor explained that the brain was a complicated organ, with a tremendous amount of loops and branches to help it process information. As an anology of BI imagine if a large city such as New York was devastated by an earthquake. If you wanted to get across town you would find bridges down and fallen buildings blocking your way. You would be able to reach your destination but it would require a lot more time. You might have to retrace your steps because of fallen debris or lack of a bridge. Dr Ryder also likened BI to a damaged telephone exchange. If someone broke into it with a rake, and swept the rake through the wires and disconnected a whole city block, this would have far-reaching ramifications.

Postscript: The Wild Goose Chase

BI was like this. Communication is scrambled, and the brain is taxed trying to understand; what had been easy and automatic is now very difficult.

He spoke of the way the BI disrupts how we process information. Brain-injured people may not feel comfortable; things such as stirring a cup of tea may no longer be automatic; they may make errors; be forgetful; or drop or spill things, which may make them feel foolish and lose self-esteem.

His golden eggs of advice on recovery included:

- Putting in effort – the more effort you put in the more you will recover. You need to adapt, to learn new tricks, to retrain.
- The brain holds off other information so that you can concentrate. BI impairs the ability to remember: if you can't find the keys, it's not that you don't remember, it's because the brain doesn't encode.
- You must slow down, use your brakes so that you become aware and do things carefully.
- Relaxation is important. Noise irritates and makes you angry, and this leads to stress. You need to focus inwardly, monitor yourself, become more aware of what's going on, become aware of strengths and personal resources.
- You need to build up your brain – recognise the things that have gone and the things that you have.
- BI will be a lifelong problem. You need the support of family, friends and a good doctor.
- Memory needs the ARM technique: Association (visualise something that has links, try to find associations), Repetition

(repeat it, say it out loud, write it, read it, listen to yourself say it), Modality (different modes or methods – such as writing, speaking and reading).
- Memory is composed of Observation (perceiving), Processing (encoding information in the brain) and Recall. Practice helps.
- The brain will sprout new fibres with use. It will slowly regrow.
- You must never give up. Don't give up, work on it, look for new handles.
- Things don't look so dark – you can move on to a more fulfilling life.

The next speaker was Deborah Fedor. What a woman! Deborah had BI, which she likened to being plucked from Brooklyn and put in Greenland. She couldn't read, she got lost when she left the house, she'd had marriage communication problems. Deborah spoke of general myths about BI – that people with BI can't think and that they're not intelligent.

Her golden eggs of advice on recovery included:

- Going outside rehab to improve: she'd gone to a nearby gym six days a week, she and her husband saw a marriage guidance counsellor who didn't know about BI but could help them with their communication problems.
- Self-talk to self-monitor.
- Be involved. BI needs work for the rest of your life. You need to develop charms, talents and improvise.
- BI is an attack on who you are. You need to find who you are again. To survive, you must do things differently.

Postscript: The Wild Goose Chase

- Everyone tries to latch on to the person before the accident – the ego gets in the way. You have to let go, experience grief then rebuild yourself using different pieces.
- You must take care of the body and take vitamin C.
- It takes time.
- You need patience and an understanding spirit. The mental and physical must be taken into account for a holistic approach.

Deborah formed the Independent Living Center, where self-help, consumer control and peer approach is part of the paradigm. She said rehab views the individual with BI as a client to be managed, fixed to fit into society. At the Center the participants control what is going on; they are given the 'dignity of risk'.

Adaptive and inventive, Center members would go to the participants' home to make helpful suggestions. For example, in one case, a gentleman was going to be put in a home because he would go out of his apartment and leave the stove on, and there was a considerable risk of fire. A solution to the problem was found by placing a light near the front door and connecting it so that it flashed if the stove was left on. The man would see the flashing light when he wanted to leave, and be reminded to turn off the stove. (Similar lights are used by people who cannot hear, to alert them to audible signals.)

Another example: a doctor with BI was fading away from lack of food. They found countless jars of salad dressing in her apartment. Apparently she'd be overwhelmed when in the supermarket, grab some salad dressing and flee. Using the peer approach where BI people help each other, a map of the supermarket was drawn up and inside the door of her pantry was a list of food, shelves to place them on, and tick lists to complete.

The Independent Living Center has a firm belief that you should do what you want to do, be what you want to be.

One sunny afternoon later that week Ted and I admired the flowers and skaters at Rockefeller Centre. We walked on through Central Park in the sunshine, watching squirrels dancing amid the leaves, and sparrows cheekily taking grain from between the hooves of the horses lined up with their carriages. Further along a dog-walker passed, with half a dozen dogs of various breeds on leads harmoniously leading the way (were all dogs in New York on Mogadon?). Eventually we reached the marble halls of Mount Sinai Hospital and were ushered into Dr Gordon's room. Ted and I felt honoured that such an eminent person would give us his time.

'What can I do for you?' he asked, somewhat professionally.

'I want the golden keys that unlock the door to set free the brain-injured person.' I was shaking inside. What a stupid thing to say. We'd travelled halfway round the world to ask such a famous and eminent person such a question. Beside me I could sense Ted groaning inwardly, thinking, 'Now she's done it!'

To our relief my request was met with a warm smile.

His golden eggs of advice for recovery:

- Remember that the process of trying to constantly reconcile who you were, who you are and who you want to be never ends.
- Don't give up hope.

Postscript: The Wild Goose Chase

- Be relentless.
- Realise that more is being found out about BI. The past fifteen years have been concentrated on survival for people with BI. Research is indicating there are health-related issues with BI: endocrine and pituitary dysfunction, body changes, colds, flu, respiratory difficulties, continence problems etc.
- Write everything down.
- Realise there is no golden pill to make you better.
- Never give up.

Dr Gordon then took us personally to visit the new Mount Sinai Rehabilitation wing and explained what was being done. Such kindness was most touching.

We walked back through Central Park as the stars came out in a prussian blue sky and a half-moon hung above the lit Chrysler Building. Our last night in the Big Apple. Somewhere over the rainbow we had flown and found greater happiness, knowledge and understanding.

Waiting for breakfast the next morning I picked up a newspaper, the one and only one I had tried to read during our short trip. An article entitled 'Music and strong spirit carry pianist past adversity' caught my attention. Ana Maria Trenchi Bottazzi was to play her fourteenth concert at Carnegie Hall that night. In 1961 her car ploughed into a truck on an icy road. A surgeon removed fifteen blood clots and replaced her forehead with a platinum plate. But he could not replace her energy, her coordination or her ability to recall pages of music. Those qualities took years of working through. The pain initially prevented her from striking a single piano key.

Doing Up Buttons

She never believed the surgeon who said she would not perform again. After thirteen years of recovering her physical and mental abilities, Bottazzi returned to the concert stage, with a repertoire of three thousand pieces from memory. She has been awarded the All Nations' Women's League Woman of the Year in 1982, a United Nations award as an outstanding person in 1984, and the New York Governor's outstanding achiever's award in 1993.

As our plane soared over New York I could just imagine her music soaring around Carnegie Hall. *We can fly*.

MAKING HEADWAY

Some Thoughts on Change

Have you ever plugged in the hair-drier or the toaster when the switch to the electricity supply was on? Did you have a tiny thrill, a surge of 'Phew, it didn't get me, I've cheated death'? Perhaps we constantly flirt with death to reinforce the feeling that we are immortal, that death will pass us by. We rarely, if ever, wonder what we would do, how we would cope or imagine what would become of us if we were to get badly injured and our whole life were to be changed.

Loss

We say it's good to change our socks, yet bad to change our minds. We spend quite a lot of our time planning change: that new outfit, a longed-for trip, a desired extension to our house. Most people believe that it is normal practice to resist change. But do we? Do we resist a pay rise? Do we resist replacing the broken fridge? No. The degree of resistance to change depends on the type of change involved, and how well it's understood. What people resist is not change but loss, or the possibility of loss.

We're most likely to resist change when we lose the known or tried, and we're concerned over the personal loss of something already gained. Change threatens the 'investment' we have made in the status quo, and is often difficult to come to terms with.

I have not only been trying to come to terms with pain but also with a total change in every aspect of my life, from the most personal moments to coping with others to how they cope with the changes in me. I am trying to come to terms with the profound loss of who I was and all that I had worked so hard to achieve.

Doing Up Buttons

Acting

Very early on in my recovery two facts became glaringly apparent. The first was that people found it difficult to cope with a 'changed' person, which meant that I 'acted' to pretend that massive changes had not taken place. Why? To make them feel comfortable. The second fact was that because I still looked the same, people were further confused – they simply could not understand that life was no longer the same for me. Once again, acting was important. Now perhaps acting has a positive side, as the old song says, 'Whenever I feel afraid I hold my head erect, and whistle a happy tune so no-one will suspect I'm afraid . . . and I fool myself as well'.

Even the 'experts', rehab people, appear to have difficulty recognising or coming to grips with the fact that their 'patients' used to have full, happy and busy lives before their accidents. They used to be people before they were patients; too often this does not seem to be acknowledged. The charade continues, with the inference that life goes on in the same way. By doing that, however, we continue to reinforce such a notion, so the change gets buried deeper and deeper. Our puzzlement as to what is really wrong with us grows and we become further confused.

When I saw a certain doctor her opening words were, 'Well, you've had a lot of changes in your life recently!' Relief washed over me. Here, at last, was someone who could help me because she understood that what I was trying to do was come to terms with CHANGE.

I was trying to come to terms with change in every facet of my life: my relationship with myself, my husband, my children, my family, my friends, the doctors, and at school with colleagues and students.

Relationships with People

An unexpected 'threatening' group of people has been strangers. Perhaps in my desire to appear normal I try too hard and frequently burst into tears on the phone or when in shops in front of strangers. Then words would escape me. I need a card with the words: 'I'm sorry I have embarrassed you: I've had an accident, at times the words won't come out.'

I am no longer in control of my relationships with people, and this change has been quite frightening. I have lost so many of the skills that I had worked to develop over the last decades.

Why Me?

Another apparent and strange happening is how differently people treat you. I believe that people are more primitive and superstitious than we could ever contemplate. On initial contact they quite obviously try to find out why you had the accident – perhaps to make sure they don't make the same mistake? On learning that you made no mistake – that it was someone else's fault – several reactions begin to surface. The first contains an element of relief, as if there is only so much bad luck floating around, and if something has happened to you, there is less chance of the same happening to them. The second is the element of 'you get what you deserve', the myth that we have grown up with and absorbed from fairy stories, myths, legends and stories with a moral. The third and most upsetting is the notion that 'it is all for the best', 'it was meant to be' or 'I told you so – it will all work out well in the end.'

The frequency with which these sentiments are used would suggest that they are firmly embedded in the community as either ways of showing sympathy or as desensitising coping strategies. Unfortunately these reactions tend to further confuse, make guilty and bewilder the accident victim.

What is needed is being allowed to talk, expressions of sympathy, acknowledgement that it's dreadful and most unfair, and an offer to be of help in any way they can as they realise life will be difficult for you.

Mourning

It was quite obvious that the changes in my life led to loss and mourning. The stages of acceptance I went through were similar to those people pass through when someone has died.

As I came to in Intensive Care in hospital I was in denial, and avoided confronting reality. I can remember thinking to myself on countless occasions, 'This is not happening to me, this is a dream.'

Very gradually a new thought surfaced to challenge the denial: 'Why me?' It seems crazy that these two opposite thoughts jostled to take control of my mind.

Then came a macabre dance of realisation, awareness and waves of anguish and depression. Eventually, like the first feeble green shoots of spring through the blanket of winter's snow, came a tentative acceptance that what had happened had happened, and I was determined to make the best of the situation.

Symbols and Rituals

Rituals, ceremony, stories and symbols can be valuable tools when used with damaged persons, to assist them to come to terms with, and start to understand, their changed selves.

I needed something almost like a funeral service for the person I had been, and a thanksgiving service that I had survived and could have a second chance at life. Change MUST be acknowledged if an accident victim is to 'move on'.

Concrete symbols can be of immense advantage to help accident victims understand why they are undergoing rehabilitation. I have seen the bewilderment, confusion and downright disobedience by people at rehab classes; the unspoken or spoken cry of 'Why am I here? I just want to go home.' We have gone through so much change already: instead of our usual routine our days are now spent at doctors, having tests and having our condition noted. Change for us is unjust and abhorrent.

I have found that if I have something to hold in my hand to feel, touch and see, this symbol reminds me why I am undergoing rehabilitation. For me, a small mirror would help answer the question 'Why am I here?' A fifty-cent coin would represent my ability to earn money, to be independent and a functioning member of society. A single jigsaw puzzle piece represents my need to fit back into my life.

It's amazing that while I was in hospital my family discussed having a party to thank all the kind people involved in helping us during those early difficult weeks. This was to be a party to say 'I'm better'. After many months we did have a party to say 'I think I'm starting to feel a little better'. Ceremonies are enmeshed in the recovery process, and all need to be acknowledged and celebrated: visits, gifts, flowers, the stepping stones of upward movement from Intensive Care to ward to home to the first step unaided, the first shower and so on.

I am astounded at the satisfaction and relief I experienced after having my day in court, of being able to tell my story and see justice delivered to the person who created my pain and damage. The ritual of the court was not about the other driver getting what he deserved or being punished, but a public acknowledgement that the accident happened, that things have changed for me.

Acknowledging change enabled me to move forward to the next stage of change.

What Have Others Done?

Once I started to feel better I was consumed with desire to find out how other people have coped. I suppose I am looking for role models in this foreign land I find myself in. Stories and books written by other people who have been in my predicament have helped on so many levels, even by simply affirming the reality of my journey.

Fredrick Linge, a clinical psychologist, suffered brain damage after a car accident. He has slowly recovered most of his facilities. In Linge's own words:

> I have been on the outside looking in, and on the inside

Some Thoughts on Change

looking out of the world of the brain-damaged person. I have found that internal and external factors must mesh smoothly in order for the brain-damaged person to reach his fullest potential and cope with his disabilities ... People close to me tell me that I'm easier to live with and work with, now that I'm not the highly self-controlled person that I used to be. My emotions are more open and more accessible, partly due to the brain damage that precludes any storing up of emotions, and partly due to the maturational aspects of this whole life-threatening experience. I have come through the crisis of my life with more respect for myself and others.

Tony Moore's book *Cry of the Damaged Man* tells of one man's struggle to return to life after a horrific car crash. A couple of months after my accident the mother of one of my students brought me a copy. I read it frantically, with incredible difficulty, with eyepatch and ruler, searching in every page for hope, hope that he would return to 'normal' and that life for him had not really changed. My realisation that his life was profoundly altered seven years after the accident threw me into the bitterest despair. I am only now facing the fact that I am a different person from before the accident. Accepting change is the most important pivot, and affects all of recovery from an accident. In 'Personal Changes' Moore says:

> I changed because of the accident. Some of the alterations were the directly enforced effects of the injuries. But the significant ones began during the time when my spirits reached rock bottom. The months of recovery provided

Doing Up Buttons

> the time for the changes to build their own strength.
>
> For me change was an extended process, not an event ...
>
> The feeling which returned again and again was one of alteration. At first, the changes were all reductions. I felt that life had become restrained and restricted so that a sense of loss touched everything. The accident altered my opportunity to do the things which gave me pleasure and altered the pleasure provided by the things I was still able to do.

Oliver Sacks' book *The Man Who Mistook His Wife for a Hat* gave me immeasurable comfort. I was transfixed, and 'consumed' this book in a single day, hardly able to tear myself away from the pages long enough to eat. So many of the chapters spoke to me, for instance, 'The man who mistook his wife for a hat'. How frequently have I also mistaken things! Did this explain why the green traffic light meant 'drop your handbag' and not 'cross the road'?

Another chapter, 'The disembodied lady', suggested the reason why I walked into walls, forgot to dry my left leg, knocked things over and bashed and burnt my left side.

'The dog beneath the skin' let me feel more normal about my heightened sense of smell for a few weeks when – on doctor's orders – I coped without the eyepatch with gross double vision (the vision was so confusing I preferred to go about with my eyes closed).

Sacks states that the patient's essential being is very relevant in the higher reaches of neurology and in psychology; for here the patient's personhood is essentially involved, and the study of disease and identity cannot be disjointed. We may say they

Some Thoughts on Change

are travellers to unimaginable lands, lands of which otherwise we should have no idea or conception. A section of tales is entitled 'Losses'. By reading of these changes in others lives one does not feel so isolated as a member of the human race.

Cooperation and Communication

Rehab personnel seem to overestimate the degree of cooperation they will get from the patient. May I suggest that among the many reasons for this lack of cooperation is confusion? Patients have nothing in their experience to assist them to know what to do in the strange predicament they have found themselves. Not knowing what is required of them is disempowering. In many instances they may feel like 'lesser beings', their lives having been taken over by all-knowing experts.

Family and friends are perhaps equally at sea, so one has to rely on the experts. Unfortunately experts are often too busy to explain what is happening and why certain procedures are applied. Patients need to be empowered, to feel that they have some say in their rehabilitation process. We need to be asked 'What do you feel your main needs are?' We need to feel that our voices have been heard, not simply objects for the experts to judge and assess.

Patients need explanations for why certain things are done. Tasks need to be explained: 'Today we will tackle these skills. They will help you with . . . I will be watching to make sure you achieve this . . . and that.'

We need a curriculum, not just a timetable. We need a simple, clear, precise, well-ordered, indexed, user-friendly booklet that explains who does what, with a space for our own personal occupational therapist's name etc – this could be a sticker that is inserted as required. We need to know who tackles what, and a brief description of how the problem is tackled.

Mentor Figure

I am not a client, a resident or a patient.
I am a person, a citizen, an individual.
I have value and worth – recognize this!
— *Independent Living Center, New York*

A 'control' or 'mentor' figure who oversees the whole program would be a great advantage. BI people need to be given responsibility so they can cooperate and play a more active and positive part in learning how to handle the process of change. Rehabilitation is like a school that prepares people for the life that was their own, that somehow has been taken away from them.

BI people may be suffering from 'overload', trying to come to terms with change in every aspect of their lives, from the basics of walking, talking and thinking, to learning everything anew. The complexity of even the simplest tasks means that everything needs to be broken down into manageable pieces.

Managers and leaders are crucial in helping the BI person. Managers wield authority, reorganise, think logically, consider dangers, formulate policies, take charge, scrutinise performance and instruct. Leaders apply influence, rethink, think laterally, sense opportunities, set examples, let go, search for potential and inspire.

This person has a vital part to play when 'managing' the changes in the patient's life. He or she needs to be both manager and leader, to keep one eye on managing the patient, and the other on establishing direction, communication and energy.

Incompatibility

Incompatibility can be a major problem between the patient and the rehab personnel. With the patient in a state of heightened emotions during the adjustment period, friction can be unbearable. I have found it is impossible to learn from someone who did not appear to like or value me. When a patient is having difficulty or avoiding doing something he or she needs to do, it may be because the rehab person has not presented the steps to be taken in a positive, sensible, helpful manner. Body language and tone are all important. Compatibility is crucial in the delicate process of enabling the patient to accept change.

Having Something to Do

If someone asked me what helped me turn the corner of black despair I'd have to answer doing tapestry. It must have been a year after the accident, and I was obviously feeling bored and frustrated, when Ann suggested that I try to do a little on the tapestry I had taken on the plane to Mexico. The thought that I had held and stitched it when my life was so different made me feel I could somehow recapture the past or at least remember. I had a burning desire to finish a tapestry for Rob's

Doing Up Buttons

twenty-first. So with eyepatch and basket of wools by my side, I picked up the half-finished canvas.

Tapestry had long been a pleasurable part of my life. I'd moved on from large printed canvases of the 'Lady and the Unicorn' and copies of the Bayeaux Tapestries for Helen, Ann and Ken's twenty-firsts to 'painting' in wool after scribbling on a blank canvas with Texta. One of the earliest thoughts that flashed through my mind when I felt I was dying was 'But I haven't done Rob's twenty-first tapestry yet'. Perhaps so many hundreds of hours had been spent on tapestries for the others that I had a really firm desire to accomplish this!

I still had double vision for reading on white paper but my hands could feel where the holes were. I had discovered something I could do to help fill in the long hours.

It is such an old and hackneyed expression but it is true in many ways – 'time is a great healer'. It is not time itself but how we use it to learn and grow and cope that makes us heal, both mentally and physically. The painful lessons, coping strategies devised, acceptance and expectations eventually settle into more realistic reality. But do we make our own reality or does reality make us?

Small Can Be Big

Perceptions are of prime significance. Let me share a story my physio told me. Phillip thrived on sailing his yacht in races. One Saturday he won his first race with flying colours. The second race of the day was a dangerous disaster. The weather was the same, the crew was the same, the yacht was the same but not quite – the small linchpin in the tiller was different –

Some Thoughts on Change

his young daughter had lost the old one after the last race so he inserted a new pin but did not bend it. The pin fell out and was lost overboard. The tiller became useless and they could not steer the boat. Just a slight bend in a pin – such a small component of the entire sailing experience – yet so important and devastating is its loss.

This story brought home to me how small things can have big consequences, how small changes to our lives can have long-lasting consequences.

The changes in a person's life may appear similar in proportion to the bend in the linchpin: infinitesimal in scale, but capable of devastating results.

Doing the Right Thing at the Time

A friend's husband had a severe stroke, and for many years, she nursed and helped him, often perplexed by the crazy things this once-brilliant man did. One afternoon he was missing for several hours. She searched everywhere for him, and eventually found him down the back garden, sitting in the disused outside toilet. He had a rubbish bin on his knees and fifteen neckties round his neck. After she managed to extract him from his predicament she asked him, 'Why did you do it Dick? Why?' The reply of this formerly brilliant man, whose damaged brain at times let him see things with crystal clarity was, 'Because it seemed like a good idea at the time.'

When we look back on how we've tried to handle the past and how we've coped, perhaps all we do is answer like Dick: at the time it seemed a good idea. We need to keep this in

Doing Up Buttons

mind when examining strange coping strategies of ourselves and others.

Being Alone

Another different and unexpected experience after being in an accident is learning to live with yourself. One tends to forget that one's entire life has been busy and spent reacting with others: at school, when studying, working, with a young family etc. There was always a focus in life and interaction with others. But an accident victim is suddenly cut off from life, working life and interactions. There may be few things left that can be done to distract one from thinking – personally I could not read, listen to the radio, watch TV, garden, shop or do housework. I could not communicate properly with others, and felt isolated, like an alien.

Perhaps the greatest change in my life has been coping and accepting that I would have to spend a large proportion of my time alone. This is something I've only experienced once before in my life, and that was when I were expecting Helen. Apart from the last few months of the pregnancy, most of my waking hours have been spent being busy with other people. There was never much time for reflective thinking, life was always a rush. With four kids, a full-time job, study, home and garden no sooner would one start pondering some 'big' question of life that a 'must do' would slip in to be handled.

Now my thoughts and imagination are my constant companion. Having to go 'cold turkey' and manage without the substance that gives you a buzz is difficult. Distractions as varied as working, planning, working towards the future,

Some Thoughts on Change

constant contact with people, to always having something that needed doing are gone. Work and people had given me my buzz in the past. Loneliness, or being on one's own for long periods of time, is hard to get used to.

I thought that I would solve these problems by helping stroke victims. I completed the training at the hospital in a daze. When I was allotted a person to visit, I caught a taxi to his home, only to discover that he was in a much better state than I was. So I decided to conserve my strength.

Concentrating on small pleasures can help. So, in another way, small can become big. Things that in normal life would be taken for granted or dismissed in a second can add richness and meaning to life.

Optimism needs to be cultivated with positive self-talk and self-pats on the back. The overwhelming feelings of helplessness, frustration and failure can be pushed to one side if you can find something that you can do to get a sense of achievement, whether it be setting the table or finding someone YOU can help. I remember telling myself that feeling bad and sorry for myself were luxuries I couldn't afford!

Excuses aplenty abound when you are trying to push yourself to do something difficult or that you feel you might fail at. But effort and energy are necessary to push yourself to do more.

One thing that is certain is that things change. No matter how you feel at the moment, no matter how low or worthless you feel, you must keep in mind that your feelings will change.

🥀 Game-playing

People play games. We all know that but the games people play make coming to terms with change even harder to cope with. 'Good manners' can make it impossible to really say how you feel.

'Unwritten rules' regulate how we communicate with people and what the 'done' thing to do is. For example, how often do we answer 'I'm fine' when in fact we feel lousy?

🥀 Communication: Speaking and Listening

I realise now that there are many little tools I could have used to help myself if only I had known about them or had the capacity to ask someone to help. Those who have suffered head injury or trauma may have difficulty speaking or understanding. We all take it totally for granted that we can speak and express our ideas and someone will understand us, or if they don't quite 'get' what we're saying they can ask questions to find out.

Can you imagine how you'd feel if you couldn't find the words or understand even simple requests? To be unable to pick up and understand non-verbal clues: body language, gestures and facial expressions, all those things that help us interpret and understand words. Add to this short-term memory loss, when you can't remember what the topic of the conversation is, and communication becomes a hit-and-miss affair that is difficult and perplexing. All these only further isolate the head-injured person.

Speaking is a complicated process, perhaps a bit like making

Some Thoughts on Change

pancakes. First you have to have a recipe (you need a thought and desire to impart it to someone). You then go to the pantry to assemble all the ingredients (you need to select the right words from all the words you know). Next, you assemble the ingredients in the right order (you assemble the words using the right grammar), then pour the mixture into the pan and turn the pancake over (you select the right sounds to make individual words and use the right muscles from your diaphragm, throat, jaw, tongue and lips to make the sentence). Simple? No!

Understanding is a complex process: from hearing and remembering the complete sentence, to understanding the meanings of the individual word, to linking it all together to understand what has been said. It's a bit like translating from another language. At times you get stuck on translating or understanding an individual word, get lost, and forget what was said. It is very important to establish the topic of discussion from the beginning. When the BI listener is made aware of the topic – for instance, cars or holidays – they can tune into the vocabulary. A filing drawer in their mind is open at the right location. This can help with guessing or understanding the words in context.

Speaking is equally complex. From the thought you wish to impart you then select the correct vocabulary. Frequently you get stuck trying to find the right word – actions or telling about the topic can help the listener to guess or understand.

Communication problems can vary depending on the area or areas of the brain affected. Difficulties can be slight to severe. *Dysarthria* occurs when the area of the brain that controls speaking is damaged, leading to a lack of coordination of muscles needed for speech. *Dyspraxia* is where there is difficulty in muscle movements involved in speech. *Dysphagia* is when there is difficulty swallowing. It was wonderful to learn that things were real, and that they had names.

I think if someone had prepared photocopied sheets with information about my problems, and put them in a slim folder for me to read, I wouldn't have been so worried. I was told to get a notebook – but at the time I wasn't even capable of organising myself. I was sufficiently anti-social to angrily reject anyone's suggestion if they had judged me and then decided that I needed help with certain things – without asking me what my difficulties were. I was so intent on proving them wrong that I couldn't modify my actions or learn anything.

A personal book would be useful if it was organised like a diary. It could be full of helpful information plus a record of things to be done. This could then become a checklist of achievements (small though they may be) so that when the BI person can't remember doing anything, at the end of the day there is at least a record of where the day went. Each day there could be a helpful hint to help the BI person remember how to do things, with coping strategies.

Sight

I was most fortunate to attend a lecture given by Dr Josephine Moore. As I heard her explain the incredible complexities of vision I could understand a little more why my faulty vision was driving me crazy.

The visual system is our most important sense in regard to learning, memory and recall, communication, spatiotemporal

Some Thoughts on Change

orientation, early warning system, visual-manual and visual-motor activities. Vision endows us with the unique ability to pick up subliminal perceptions or clues from our environment. These reinforce the anticipatory capabilities of our nervous systems and hence, our survival and adaptive skills.

Vision is a distance receptor; it alerts us to pleasure, danger or that which attracts our attention. The visual system gives us advanced warning of movement around us, as well as informing us about our own spatiotemporal movements, posture and balance.

Vision plays a critical role in attentive functions, and attends to that which is most important for learning, communicating, interacting with, plus adapting to our ever-changing environment. It is the sense that we use for understanding non-verbal communication. (Gesture or non-verbal 'language' comprises about 70 per cent of all communication between individuals, or their pets, while only 30 per cent is actual verbal language.) Visual-manual skills or eye-hand coordination, along with our amazing brains, have endowed us with the exceptional ability to continually create, invent and discover new things.

The most valuable insight I gained from attending Jo's lecture was a comment she made, in passing, about 'down-and-outers'. People who can't understand what they see down and out. This explained my difficulty recognising things in front of my face unless I knelt down and saw them level with my eyes. I was not mad. I was a 'down-and-outer'!

Doing Up Buttons

🙵 Adapting Things

It's so boring and soul-destroying to have to re-learn skills you learnt as a child, but take it as a challenge: be an inventor, use things for other purposes and do things differently. Innovation is crucial in finding ways to cope. Don't forget where there's a will, a way can be found. Head-injured people need to be active participants in learning to cope anew; they need to be interested, enticed and captivated to try and invent things to help themselves.

I realise now I passed through several stages in adapting. Like the stages of grieving, I presume some people might pass through the stages more quickly than others, while some emphasise one stage more than others. The key is to adapt things at your own speed. Take as an example setting the table.

For forty-five years I had set the table without thinking. I could do it while watching television, cooking a meal, talking on the phone and planning a lesson for the following day. Now I couldn't do it even when I gave it my whole attention. I felt an idiot.

I had no way of tackling the issue because I could not work out what I was doing wrong. Slowly, I realised that I had to examine the whole table-setting process, and break the task into several steps. I had to remember what food was to be eaten, how many people were to sit at the table, where the knives and forks were, what knives and forks looked like. I had not realised how complicated the process is if you have difficulty remembering or recognising things. I had to learn to do it all again. I must confess that after five years this is still a difficult task.

Some Thoughts on Change

I tried writing labels 'soup spoon' and 'knife', and stuck them in the cutlery drawer. I tried counting out and placing five forks or five spoons on the bench, then take them over to the table. If I'd forgotten a spoon, by the time I got back to the drawer, I'd forget what I'd come for. At this stage I was constantly trying to evaluate what was working best, and trying it out to find the way to set the table, and set steps to follow in future. Ann was a great help, reminding me patiently of steps and suggestions, and helped to write a sheet 'How to set the table'. The support and encouragement of family and friends were crucial.

This may sound like the answer to the problem, but first you had to remember you had a problem so that you could take steps to correct it. Frequently I would try to set the table the 'old' way and end up perplexed and frustrated. I'd forgotten I'd forget.

Photocopied tick-off lists for me to check before leaving the house are invaluable. I keep the piece of paper in my pocket to refer to if I suddenly think I didn't turn off the oven. I must confess that I have had to return home by taxi to check things just in case I wasn't concentrating and ticked something off the list and didn't check it. So now, as well as ticking things on a list, I place articles near the stove or iron, say, an onion or a ball. I say to myself stove/onion, iron/ball. When I write onion/ball, I remember I have checked things. These lists are a good habit.

Many useful things have helped me: a long-handled shoe horn to stop my ribs poking out when I bend over, a very long handle on the broom and rake so that I can put my arm up and get some force, hot packs to put in the microwave, a lightweight electric blower to get rid of leaves on the path, a cordless, portable phone, building metre-high walls into the slope, thus making raised garden beds so that I can weed without bending down, and a lightweight metal trolley to carry things when shopping.

In many different ways I tried to be innovative in solving problems. But the more I did, the more problems there were to solve! It was – and is – a very slow process.

Worries

All too frequently when we're frustrated with worries we can't think of what to do to help to relieve the pressure. Here is an alphabet of suggestions. Try choosing one suggestion and adapting it to your situation.

Appreciate something.
Bawl: have a good cry.
Call up a friend.
Drink a coffee.
Escape from it with a movie, TV or story.
Fight for your rights: focus on something.
Go away from where you are, even for a night.
Hope is worth hanging on to. Home is a sanctuary and sweet, be happy.
Invest in friends and the future.
Jealousy can ruin our lives. Recognise it, deal with it.
Knit, sew, do things with your hands.
Laugh.
Make things happen.

Nothing stays the way it is, remember this.
Observe how others have coped.
Pray and or plan for something.
Question.
Run, walk, be physical.
Spoil yourself.
Talk about it.
Understand your condition.
Very positive attitudes help.
Walk it away.
e**X**orcise the demons lurking inside by bringing them out into the light.
Yell, curse, let off steam.
Zzz – sleep.

Happiness

I've thought about happiness, and what constitutes happiness. What makes a happy person? The traits of happy people seem to be self-esteem, optimism, extroversion and personal control. No wonder my happiness was gone for so many years. No self-esteem, nothing to look forward to, inability to be friendly due to my difficulty with communication, and absolutely no personal control. If only I had been aware of how disempowering my circumstances were, I would not have felt bad, or stupid and ungrateful that I was not happy.

I have learnt to enjoy the present because happiness is not a date in the future, nor is the present only a way to get to the future. I have learnt to live and enjoy each moment rather than thinking ahead all the time.

Doing Up Buttons

There have been many frightening, disappointing and sad events during the last five years. Feelings of isolation and powerlessness would dump on me, like a massive wave, often when I least expected them.

There was the evening of the terrible storm. Ted was overseas, I was marooned on my hillside and Rob had not returned home from school. I tried ringing all his friends but no-one knew of his whereabouts. There were two ways he could return home, each in opposite directions. If he'd caught the train he would have had a two-kilometre rain-swept walk along unmade back roads, lanes and some paddocks. The other way was up the hill from the bus. I was frantic. If I could have driven I would have driven round the streets in search of him. I clearly remember grabbing my walking stick, coat and soggy eyepatch and wandering around the hilltop in the storm, hoping to see him. When eventually I walked straight into him in the lane by the paddock, I was beside myself.

Having an accident has not been a happy experience!

Having An Accident is Not All Bad

My accident has led me to a deeper appreciation of life, family and friends. It has given me time to reflect on life, and I hope that maybe others can learn from my experiences. Employment for doctors, physios, occupational therapists, taxi-drivers, housecleaners and other teachers at school have been generated.

The importance of small things cannot be overestimated. Memories like faded forgotten rose petals found in a drawer need revisiting. Photos are needed to bring back the colour.

Some Thoughts on Change

Questions abound. We obviously have to help ourselves but how can we do that? Who can help us? What can be done to forget the whole episode? Is it just a matter of time healing and new pleasant experiences flowing in to dilute the bad ones? Do you need to be selfish to be kind? Do you need to focus on what makes you more comfortable, which is the opposite of how you used to put others first in your previous lifestyle?

If everyone appears to have four eyes, which they don't in reality, what is real? Can I believe my eyes? Where do memories go? What is really real?

THE TEN COMMANDMENTS FOR
COPING

1. TRY TO HAVE SOME CONTROL OVER YOUR TIME

Remember fatigue will get you and make concentration very difficult. Make a structured routine. Have a set sequence for each day (this will help your memory and help to reduce stress). A calm, well-organised environment really helps. Accept that you may only have one hour's 'good' time a day. The morning when you are fresh may be a good time to achieve things; try to accomplish something then. From experience you can't expect the 'good' time to expand quickly. I have found that it is about an hour a year. At five years I only have four or five productive hours a day. This is broken into three hours in the morning and a couple of hours after my afternoon nap.

2. HAVE ORDER IN YOUR DAY

Prioritise. Break tasks into separate chunks. Write things down. Take notes during conversations so you can follow the discussion. I find that preparing notes in point form helps me cope with situations at home and at work.

3. DON'T BITE OFF MORE THAN YOU CAN CHEW

Have reasonable expectations and don't be discouraged if mistakes happen. Everybody makes mistakes. Don't blame others or yourself for mistakes.

Some Thoughts on Change

4. Don't get the guilts
Don't feel guilty if things do not work out. Remember you will 'get lost' in conversations as well as places. It's OK!

5. Don't work at it all day
Do something that you like each day (it might be something like ringing a friend or sitting in the sun having hot chocolate or watching TV). Find something each day to be pleased about or thankful for (try to concentrate on finding something worthwhile).

6. Try to do something to help someone else
Try to help your family each day. This will make you feel better and less of a burden. Little tasks like setting the table or unpacking the dishwasher do make a difference to all.

7. Don't give in
Tell yourself when the going gets tough the tough get going, and if at first you don't succeed try and try again. There is no failure except in no longer trying.

8. Don't think things should be simple
Try to see that there are problems you are trying to contend with: physical pain and difficulties, finding out about head damage and learning to cope and work around the difficulties, emotional healing, coping with grief and loss, learning to know yourself and your limitations, and trying to have confidence in yourself as an individual.

9. Don't diversify

Remember to simplify if you have a one-track mind. Reason in a straightforward manner rather than try to cope with complex issues.

10. Try to eliminate distractions

Noise and chaos make it hard to absorb information. The more distractions around me, the less I am able to cope. For parties and family gatherings I find I can cope better on a one-to-one basis in a separate room rather than in with the mob.

HELP SECTION

The Brain and Brain Injury
Based on information from Headway Victoria

What is brain injury?

Brain injury includes: Acquired Brain Damage (ABD), Traumatic Brain Injury (TBI), Head Injury (HI), Acquired Cerebral Insult (ACI), Alcohol Related Brain Injury (ARBI).

The brain is complex – it controls everything we do. If it is injured the problems for the person varies depending on which part of the brain is damaged, and how severe the damage is. ABD is a major cause of permanent disability in Australia. If you are in the 16–24 age group there is a 1 in 200 chance of acquiring brain injury. In Australia 320 000 people suffer from brain injury. If neurological diseases are added to the list, the number of people swells to 570 000.

In the fifth year after my accident Headway Victoria, an association set up to support people who have sustained head injury, produced an information kit. Knowledge is power. Just learning about HI made me feel like a normal person with HI and not a mad person. ABD, particularly as a result of road accidents, is a recent worldwide 'epidemic'.

Head-injured people experience changes in the way they think, feel and act. They may have difficulty remembering names or new information, or may become more easily upset or angry, and they may have trouble starting or finishing jobs. Any of these changes can make life very difficult at home, at school and at work. Family and friends are also affected.

Neuro-psychological rehabilitation is a comparatively new

field. It is directed specifically at rehabilitation of people who have sustained brain injury, and it addresses a vast array of cognitive and psychological disturbances. Coping with the effects of cognitive, emotional and psychological change requires positive psychological adjustment. This is the most important aspect of the rehabilitation process. The person feels a loss of self-confidence, an inability to cope, coupled with anxiety and concern about potential for recovery.

Many people do not begin to accept that they have residual cognitive and psychological problems until sufficient time has passed for them to come to terms with the fact that the disturbances in thinking and behaviour are likely to be permanent. Change is a process, not an event, and coping with change takes time.

The *Journal of Head Trauma Rehabilitation* publishes up-to-date findings of how to treat people thus afflicted. I was delighted to read that it suggests that rehabilitation teams should:

- Capitalise on the clients' strengths rather than focus on their weaknesses.
- Fully involve clients in the development of strategies.
- Ensure understanding by clients of the potential value of the technique.
- Regularly monitor the effectiveness and value of strategies as conditions change.
- Introduce strategies gradually.

The *Journal of Applied Rehabilitation Counselling* emphasises that there are changes that may affect intelligence, perception,

The Brain and Brain Injury

memory, learning, thinking and reasoning. Rehabilitation services to deal with severe traumatic brain injury are often inadequate, and undue attention is frequently placed on the physical disabilities, with little attention given to the psychological and social consequences. Physical weakness, spasticity and dysphasia tend to show eventual improvement, whereas the effects on brain injury on the client's intellectual, cognitive, social and emotional functioning are often the cause of serious and lasting disability.

After much searching through rehabilitation literature I am amazed that coping with change does not feature strongly as an integral part of rehabilitation of the individual.

We can close our eyes to imagine what it would be like to be blind. We can perhaps imagine coping with life in a wheelchair, but brain damage and the changes it brings are so difficult to perceive. We need to be aware of the impact and all encompassing nature of this, the 'king of change'.

What is traumatic brain injury?

Traumatic brain injury (TBI) is damage to the brain caused by a blow to the head or by the head being forced to move rapidly forward or backward, usually with some loss of consciousness. This may be the result of a motor vehicle accident, sports accident, gunshot wound or violent shaking (particularly of a young child). As a result of this blow or rapid movement the brain may be torn, stretched, penetrated, bruised or become swollen. Oxygen may not be able to get through to the brain cells and there may be bleeding.

The effects of TBI can be temporary or permanent, and can range from mild injury, such as may result from being momentarily stunned while playing football, to very severe injury, such as may result from a head-on car crash causing prolonged loss of consciousness. Anyone who has been concussed for any period of time, however slight the impact, may have some brain damage. While most people make a good recovery, for many this damage will result in lasting effects which, even if minor, may have significant consequences.

ACQUIRED BRAIN DAMAGE

The brain can also be damaged as a result of a stroke, alcohol, infection and disease, near-drowning, haemorrhage, AIDS and other disorders such as Parkinson's disease, multiple sclerosis and Alzheimer's disease. The terms acquired brain damage (ABD) or acquired brain injury (ABI) are used to describe all types of brain damage, including TBI, which occur after birth.

TBI is not the same as intellectual disability. People with brain injuries usually retain their intellectual abilities but have difficulty controlling, coordinating and communicating their thoughts and actions. Intellectual disability occurs from birth whereas TBI is acquired later. People with TBI can experience significant recovery and their treatment differs from that used for people with intellectual disability.

HOW DOES THE BRAIN WORK?

The brain controls and coordinates everything we do: thinking, breathing, walking, talking, feeling hungry, liking some things and not others, feeling angry or sad, as well as what goes on inside our bodies. It is made up of billions of nerve cells through which messages are transmitted by a combination of electrical and chemical activity. This soft, jelly-like

The Brain and Brain Injury

mass sits inside the skull, where it is suspended and cushioned by the cerebra-spinal fluid, which circulates around it and through its holes.

If you have a head injury it is helpful and interesting to learn about the different functions of the brain and have some idea of which area or areas are probably affected by the injury. When I was undergoing rehab I was desperate to find out where my brain was injured. I needed to try to make sense of some of the strange unexplained difficulties I was experiencing.

Headway literature has helped me understand about the brain. The brain is divided into a number of parts, all of which are designed to work together in harmony, much like an orchestra. The more coordinated and in tune they are with each other, the better the performance. Different parts of the brain control different functions.

The largest part of the brain is divided into two halves, which are joined in the middle. These are called the left and right hemispheres.

The left hemisphere is involved in speech, language, reasoning and logic, the rational, the objective. The right hemisphere is involved in visual information, drawing, musical appreciation, intuition, the emotional and the subjective.

The two hemispheres of the brain

LEFT HEMISPHERE	RIGHT HEMISPHERE
Right-hand control	Left-hand control
Analytic	Intuitive
Analyses the data	Responds to the data intuitively

Doing Up Buttons

LEFT HEMISPHERE	RIGHT HEMISPHERE
Logical	Spontaneous
Uses logic in handling information	Handles information spontaneously
Temporal	Atemporal
Is aware of time – past, present, future	Processes information without consideration of time
Sequential	Random
Deals with events and actions sequentially	Deals with events and actions randomly
Orderly	Diffuse
Organises information	Diffuses information
Systematic and formal	Casual and informal
Deals with information and objects in a variety of systematic ways	Deals with information and objects according to the need of the moment
Linear	Holistic
Reduces whole to parts and reassembles parts to whole	Sees only the wholeness of information and objects
Verbal	Non-verbal
Processes language into meaningful communication: receptive	Responds to tones, body language and touch
Computational: uses mathematics and computations	Visuo-spatial: perceives shapes and patterns, intuitively estimates
Practical	Originative
Concerned with cause and effect	Concerned with ideas and theories
Abstract	Sensory
Has abstract-oriented cognitive functions	Has sensory-orientated functions
Factual	Visual
Uses facts	Uses imagery
Concrete	Metaphoric
Explicit, precise	Symbolic, representational

From: Clare Cherry, Douglas Godwin, Jesse Staples Hawker, Is the Left Brain Always Right? *Hawker Brownlow Education, 1993.*

The Brain and Brain Injury

Each hemisphere is divided into four lobes. Frontal lobes are used for problem-solving, planning, making judgements and abstract thinking, and for controlling emotions, impulses and aggression.

The motor strip at the back of the frontal lobes controls movement. The motor strip to the frontal lobe of the left hemisphere controls movement of the right side of the body and vice-versa.

Temporal lobes look after memory and new learning, auditory information, enjoying music, and understanding speech and how things are ordered.

Parietal lobes are involved in monitoring sensation and body position, understanding time, recognising faces, reading and judging objects in space and the ability to tell left from right.

Occipital lobes receive and interpret visual information, colour, shape, distance.

The cerebellum is located at the back and below the main hemispheres. It controls muscle coordination needed for talking, walking, writing, etc.

The brain stem leads into the spinal cord, which regulates wakefulness, breathing, temperature and heart activity.

CLOSED HEAD INJURY

This is the most common form of brain injury. It occurs when the head is struck or moved violently, but the skull and membrane lining of the brain are not broken or penetrated.

With this kind of injury, damage occurs as the jelly-like brain moves inside the skull, causing bruising, tearing and twisting throughout the brain (a bit like what happens when a bus stops suddenly and the passengers are thrown in all directions). Damage is caused by the brain hitting the inside of the skull.

OPEN HEAD INJURY
This is when the skull and membrane lining the brain have been fractured, cracked or broken so that the brain is exposed or penetrated. Considerable local damage can occur in the area of the brain immediately below the impact, as well as more widespread damage.

COMA
This is a prolonged state of unconsciousness. Immediately after a brain injury a person may be in a coma, which means they do not open their eyes or respond to things happening around them. This may last for minutes, hours, days or weeks. In general the longer the period of coma, the more likely it is that the person will have severe damage to the brain.

POST-TRAUMATIC AMNESIA
A person coming out of a coma doesn't just wake up, but will go through a gradual process of regaining consciousness. This stage of recovery is called post-traumatic amnesia (PTA) and may last for hours, days or weeks.

At this stage people often remember things that happened before the accident, but will not be able to store continuous or recent memory, that is, they will not remember what happened just a few hours or even a few minutes ago.

People in PTA are partially or fully awake, but confused about the day and time, where they are, what is happening, and sometimes who they are. They may be afraid, physically

The Brain and Brain Injury

and verbally abusive, disinterested, agitated and restless. They may hallucinate and be delusional. Too much stimulation during this time may compound their confusion and distress.

People do not usually have any memory of this period – or of the accident – afterwards. There is no point trying to force them to remember. They may later describe the experience of PTA as like being in a bad dream. As they recover some people experience 'islands' or flashes of memory about this period and the accident.

The length of PTA is frequently used as a guide to the severity of brain injury. In general, if this stage lasts for more than one week, ongoing cognitive problems may be expected.

Of each 1000 people who survive a severe brain injury:

- about two-thirds will experience good recovery but possibly with some ongoing cognitive and/or behavioural problems.
- about one-quarter will have a moderate disability.
- about 10 per cent will have a severe disability.
- only 1 per cent will be in a permanent coma-like state.

POSSIBLE CONSEQUENCES OF TRAUMATIC BRAIN INJURY

Physical deficits
- paralysis with spasticity and diminished, or loss of control, of movement and skills
- fatigue
- involuntary purposeless movements, tremors, slowness of movement and/or rigidity

Doing Up Buttons

- incoordination of movement, limb weakness
- expressive aphasia (with/without profane language)
- postural insecurities (though these probably result from sensory deficits)
- seizure disorders of all kinds.

Sensory deficits
- visual deficits of all kinds are very common
- sensory dyspraxias (difficulty performing voluntary movements – not due to weakness – but because of motor-coordination problems, problems with dressing, eating, drinking, writing etc.)
- neglect syndromes (visual, auditory, motor and combinations)
- receptive aphasia (difficulty understanding or expressing language (with/without profane language)
- global aphasia (profane language still possible)
- auditory deficits (localisation of sound in space, auditory processing problems)
- dizziness or sensations of instability, and/or postural insecurity.

Personality and behavioural deficits
- diminished, or loss of, anticipatory behaviours
- learning or re-learning problems: diminished (or loss of) ability to lay down new memories
- disorientation in time and space
- perseverative behaviours (the inappropriate persistence of a response in a current task which may have been appropriate for a former task, either verbal or motoric)

The Brain and Brain Injury

- emotional liability (hyperemotional, dull, stubborn, temperamental, and/or uncontrollable fear, anger, rage, violence continuum)
- personality changes: uncooperative, neglectful, careless, no longer loving etc.
- changes in intellect, motivation or drive, and judgement
- sleeping disorders and changes in circadian rhythms
- eating disorders
- sexual and/or moral deviations
- substance abuse
- depression and/or suicidal ideation.

In rehabilitation of the TBI patient many of the motor and sensory deficits can be minimised or improved, compensated for, or the individual may be able to adapt to the disability over time. 'Personality and behavioural deficits' constitutes the major hurdles that interfere with the success or failure of the rehab team's efforts, the individuals' support systems or care-takers and their care, and the eventual disposition of the TBI client.

WHAT PROBLEMS CAN BE EXPECTED?
Acquired brain injury is often called the 'hidden disability' because its long-term problems are usually in the areas of thinking and behaviour. These are not as easy to see and recognise as many physical disabilities. As a consequence, the difficulties people with brain injury face may be ignored or misunderstood. They may be seen, even by their friends and family, as lazy or hard to get along with. There is very little understanding and knowledge in the community about brain injury and its long-term effects.

Doing Up Buttons

The long-term effects of TBI are hard to predict and will be different for each person. In general, most people will experience increased fatigue (mental and physical) and some slowing down in the speed with which they can process information.

There are five areas in which people with brain injury may experience long-term changes:

- medical difficulties
- changes in physical and sensory abilities
- changes in ability to think and learn (cognition)
- changes in behaviour and personality (psychological)
- communication difficulties.

The extent of some of these changes – like being more impulsive or getting lost easily – may only become fully apparent after the person has been living at home for a while.

Some Common Problems of Head-damaged People
- Trouble following written directions.
- Interrupts the conversation of others.
- Tires easily.
- Has trouble following oral directions.
- Has trouble handling money.
- Makes threatening gestures.
- Is moody.
- Gets lost outside the home.
- Personal habits embarrass others.
- Cannot be relied on for truth.
- Occasionally talks about sex at the wrong times.

The Brain and Brain Injury

- Sometimes intimidates others.
- Forgets the names of people he or she sees often.
- Stands too close or too far away when talking to others.
- Uses swear words excessively.
- Sometimes lets frustration lead to anger.
- Is suspicious of others.
- Has difficulty remembering events that happened in the past 24 hours.
- Talks too loudly when talking to others.
- Occasionally acts helpless.
- Has problems remembering important things he or she must do.
- Speech is not clear.
- Often finds it difficult to make decisions.
- Talks too much.
- Tends to repeat a behaviour for no reason.
- Occasionally has verbal outbursts.
- Sometimes has physical outbursts.
- Is occasionally self-centred.
- Is sometimes impulsive.
- Is socially isolated.
- Ideas sometimes don't make sense.

From: Barry S. Willer and Richard T. Linn, Practical Issues in Behaviour Management for Family Members of Individuals with Traumatic Brain Injury

SOME PUBLIC MISCONCEPTIONS ABOUT TBI

- People believe that after several weeks in a coma, patients recognise and speak to others right away when they wake up.
- After a head injury people can forget who they are and not

recognise others, but be perfectly normal in every other way.
- Sometimes a second blow to the head can help a person remember things that were forgotten.
- A little brain damage doesn't matter since people only use part of their brains.
- How quickly a person recovers from a head injury depends mainly on how hard they work to recover.

Some Facts about Head Injury
- A person who has recovered from a head injury is less able to withstand a second blow to the head.
- Complete recovery from a head injury is not possible, no matter how badly the person wants to recover.
- People who have had one head injury are more likely to have a second one.
- After a head injury it is usually harder to learn new things than it is to remember things from before the injury.
- Even minor problems can be quite difficult for individuals and families to cope with.
- Attention to physical problems often precludes consideration of brain injury.
- The damage to the brain tends to be diffuse rather than global, affecting cognitive functions in complex ways.
- Because of the nature of nerve pathways and the interconnectedness of brain functions, the impairments are difficult to predict and can affect many different abilities.
- People need to re-learn previously known skills.
- People with BI often remember their previous skills and have difficulty in accepting their diminished abilities.

The Brain and Brain Injury

- Adjustment, coming to terms with changed circumstances and the person, drastically altered family goals, prolonged grieving and uncertainty, restructuring of the family system all are experienced with HI.
- Families experience emotions – shock, denial, anger, depression, irritability, sleeplessness, marital conflict, inability to cope, resentment, hostility, neglect, abandonment, embarrassment, fear exacerbated by lack of information and misconceptions about recovery.
- Families may lose security, predictability, future plans, control over destiny, control over caring role, privacy, finance and faith.
- There may be difficulty absorbing information in times of acute stress.
- Ways to produce an angry response: tell someone what to do, threaten someone, moralise, cite logical considerations, judge, criticise and blame, name-call, analyse, condescend, interrogate, be sarcastic, don't listen, ignore needs.
- Ways to get cooperation include: be prepared to listen, recognise the emotion, permit expression, recognise needs, negotiate, reassure, respect personal space, don't argue, be clear and firm, anticipate needs, don't ignore the person.

From: Daryl Oehm and Sandra Morris, Brainstorming: An Educational Module about Acquired Brain injury For Workers in Acute Care Settings *(Centre for Social Health/Headway Victoria, 1994).*

You, Your Lawyer and Your Court Case

In order to prepare me for the legal issues resulting from the accident, Helen spent many hours explaining some of the key issues related to the situation. Our views and my experiences may throw some light on the subject.

In Australia an injured person (plaintiff) has up to six years to issue legal proceedings against the individual who has harmed him or her (the defendant). This may seem a long period of time, however, it must be remembered that the legal process can be agonisingly slow. So, once the required period for injuries to stabilise is over it is important to see a lawyer.

With a criminal case you have no say whether or not it goes to court. The police will investigate, and take the case to court if they believe there is enough evidence to build a case. If you are the plaintiff the police will investigate. You can't have your own lawyer but the other side can. At court the barrister from the other side will cross-examine your version of the facts.

Helen has stressed that I was just a cog in the wheel. The system was not set up to punish others, and money will never compensate me for my loss. What seems important to me may not be relevant to the courts, and what seems clear now may become complex and unclear when presented by the other side. She also said that small issues which could be seen to be inconsistent can be exploited by the other side. An out-of-court settlement can be made without an admission of

You, Your Lawyer and Your Court Case

liability — that is, I could get money from the other side without them admitting they have done anything wrong. All through this, all I craved for was for Mr X to apologise.

When choosing a lawyer it is often good to start with the major law firms who specialise in the area of personal injury litigation. While there are a number of very good smaller firms, the large firms often have more expertise and the capacity to keep completely up-to-date with changes in the law in this area. You must feel comfortable with your lawyer, but it is important to remember that as a professional, he or she may not appear as sympathetic to your plight as you would like. As a lawyer, it is dangerous to get too personally involved with clients' cases as this may mar their judgement and assessment on the claim. On the other hand, if you do not like your lawyer at all or feel uncomfortable talking to him or her, it is worth searching for a more suitable and appropriate person.

At your first interview your lawyer will want to know all the details of your accident in order to assess whether or not you actually have a case. It is extremely useful to have spent some time prior to your appointment clearly writing down in chronological order the events that led to your injury, and the names and details of your major doctors. If you have other documentation such as police reports this can be useful. Before handing to your lawyer any important documentation do make sure you have a copy of it at home. While everyone is careful not to lose papers it does occur; a correlating file at home is the most sensible option.

If your lawyer advises that you do not have a case, it is essential that you listen carefully to him or her to understand the reasons why. Many individuals become extremely distressed or upset when informed that it would not be a good idea for them to litigate, and take the matter very personally. To be able to pursue a case a number of criteria need to be fulfilled, including the severity of injury and negligence. You may be terribly injured (i.e. a paraplegic) but if you cannot prove that it was another person's fault that this injury occurred, that is, through negligence, you cannot take legal action. There are other benefits available instead of suing, and it is important to listen to your options fully.

On the other hand, you may be able to clearly prove that it was another individual's fault that you were injured. However, your injuries may be deemed 'not severe' enough to warrant legal proceedings. Once again this does not mean that you are not injured or that it has not affected your life. Rather you have not qualified for the arbitrary (and often deemed draconian) threshold. If you are not satisfied with your lawyer's explanation it can be worthwhile in certain circumstances to seek a second opinion. However, after two opinions, it is advisable to confront the situation. To instigate legal proceedings on shaky foundations is a recipe for economic, emotional and physical disaster.

Litigation is a very serious business, and if a case is lost it can be very expensive and emotionally taxing. One's house, car and other assets can be used to pay legal bills in the event of an unsuccessful claim. It is very unlikely that lawyers will refuse continually to litigate your claim if it is a good one. Listen to your lawyer very carefully, request full explanations, talk about the matter with your family and friends. Do not pursue litigation against professional advice.

Once it has been decided that you are able to make a claim, you must prepare yourself and your family for a long and, at times, torturous journey. The Australian legal system is an adversarial one. This means that the other side will attempt to disprove everything you say about yourself, your injuries and the events that occurred. Simple facts you take for granted, such as the change to your lifestyle, your pain, your lack of self-esteem, will be thoroughly questioned by the defendant's solicitor. It is essential to remember throughout the whole proceeding that there are no givens in a court case. Documentation about your injuries, the impact they have had upon your lifestyle, working life, economic circumstances, family and hopes for the future will need to be submitted to the other side through your lawyers. This can be distressing as you often have to put in words only what you've thought of in your darkest hour. It can be a good idea during the early stages of recovery to keep a notebook and write down the difficulties and fears you have. It can also be useful to make sure that good photographs are taken of any scarring or other physical injuries that you may have. A strong and supportive relationship with your local GP is essential; he or she must clearly document your problems.

You will be sent to see numerous doctors, both for your own lawyers and for the other side. It is important to be honest and open, and clearly express your problems. If you are coy about your injuries and don't articulate their full impact upon your life, your case may suffer for it. On the other hand, if you exaggerate your problems and the doctors eventually discover this, your case will suffer, and your credibility and honesty will be strongly questioned in court.

Doing Up Buttons

Visiting many doctors can be frustrating, but it is part of the process, so be patient. If the time and energy spent attending doctors is bothering you, request your lawyers to re-schedule your appointments to suit. Reasonable expenses of travelling to doctors will be reimbursed to you.

At some stage during your legal proceedings your solicitor will send you to see a barrister. Just about every court case involves a barrister and a solicitor. Solicitors are the first point of contact for people taking legal action. They assess whether or not there is a valid case, take detailed statements of the incident, arrange appointments to obtain medical reports and records and issue the writ (the document that gets filed with the court and served on the other side to start the proceedings). In most cases the documents are then sent to a barrister for him/her to answer questions from the other side, called interrogates. If and when a case gets to court, it is a barrister who argues the matter before a jury and a judge. Barristers wear white wigs and black gowns in court, while solicitors can wear normal business clothes.

Like the relationship with your solicitor, it is important to feel comfortable, safe and trusting with your barrister. If you have a strong dislike of him or her, it is well within your rights to talk about finding another person to represent you. Not liking what your barrister has to say is not sufficient reason to change, rather, change if you do not like the style or personality of the chosen barrister. Try not to 'fish' around for what you want to hear.

Remember throughout your whole case that these are legal proceedings. While you should listen to the advice of the professionals you have employed, do not be afraid of asking

You, Your Lawyer and Your Court Case

questions, demanding to understand what is going on and where the proceedings are at. You are in control and should remain so.

This may mean taking family members or friend to your legal appointments if possible; it is hard to understand everything that is said to you in one go. Ask your solicitor for a list of the procedures that are going to be undertaken and approximate timing so that you can keep track of where your case is and tick off the procedures as they are completed.

Understand that long delays can occur and often, this is not necessarily the fault of your lawyers. In other cases it may be, so it is important to know what is going on. If you telephone your solicitor, you do not always need to speak to him or her personally to get an update. Very often secretaries or paralegals know the case very well and can give you a comprehensive rundown. If the paralegals are unable to answer your questions they will refer it to a solicitor. It is important to understand that what may seem urgent to you may not necessarily be so. Remember that the more often you contact your solicitor the more they will charge. Save up your questions: write them down so that when you do meet or talk with your solicitor you can cover all the issues that have been concerning you. However, if a matter is urgent, do persist in attempting to contact your legal advisers.

The law changes very quickly and often dramatically. What is good advice one year may not be the next. People often get upset or confused, believing that they have not been treated fairly. For example, years ago people who took common law cases for motor accidents received a lump sum at settlement for medical expenses. In the case of severely injured plaintiffs an award of one million dollars, which seems a huge amount, may only just allow them to survive on medication or in hospital for the rest of their life. Under certain circumstances now the Transport Accident Commission may continue paying for the medical expenses, and while a settlement for the same injury may be dramatically reduced, the outcome is basically the same. As stated previously, it is important to seek up-to-date advice from lawyers who are working in this area of the law.

A court case will never heal you. Unlike criminal litigation, a common law claim does not focus on the deeds of the defendant to prove his or her guilt. The aim of a common law case is that if you can prove that someone's actions injured you, under certain circumstances, you are entitled to economic re-imbursement for your loss of wages and loss of enjoyment of life. In many ways, the idea behind this is rather ridiculous – how can money make up for not being able to see, hear, walk or think? It cannot, but it can assist in helping you rebuild your life, find other things to do, gain dignity and, in a sense, society acknowledges that you have had a harm done to you. Understand that at the end of proceedings, even if they are successful, you will not go back to your previous way of life. Rather, you will be embarking on a long journey of learning how to build and work with what you now have physically, emotionally, and economically.

Sample Notes for Doctors' Visits

Helen helped me record regular progress reports to monitor what was wrong with me and how I coped with my various problems. These were most valuable when I went to see a doctor for assessment. I would often reply 'Fine' when they asked me how I felt, forgetting the things that were making my life miserable. I would take a list such as this when I visited a doctor. This extract was recorded two years after the accident.

Pain
There's constant pain in my back, shoulder, neck and right hip. I seem to have constant colds and muck in my chest and it's so strange, but I do a lot of involuntary sighing. At times there is extreme pain in the front from the rib fractures.

Asthma has developed in the past few months. I suspect I had my first 'attacks' earlier but I believed them to be the chest infections.

Coping: I've found that when you're in pain nothing's better than hot water: a bath, shower, spa or hot water bottle. I visit a physio once a week. I have ultrasound to the shoulder every couple of days. It's quite weird but I get creeping sensations down my affected area so it feels as if I have a knife in my back and blood is dribbling from the wound.

Due to my violent reaction to Tilcotil for epilepsy I have had to discontinue taking the drug Tegretol. This had helped greatly with pain. Painkillers don't touch the pain – and I am loath to take them – but when I'm desperate a couple of Aspro-clear help a little. If I gave in I would be quite dependent on pills.

The pain in my back has made it impossible for me to stay in bed in the morning, or rest during the day, apart from my daily afternoon nap.

Exhaustion/fatigue
Each afternoon I go unconscious and can sleep until 6 p.m. and still go to sleep at 10 p.m. What a waste of a life! Since I returned home from hospital I have been up by 8 a.m. at the latest. I now have until about 11 a.m., some days until 1 p.m., when I can cope quite well. So I now have three hours a day to 'achieve' something.

Clavicle
My clavicle has healed, but a piece of exposed bone pokes up into my shoulder. The straps of undergarments are either on one side of this silly bone, near my neck and rub on the bone, or on other side, and fall down my sloping shoulder. I have trouble with the tendons in my right arm, and at times the arm is paralysed. There's terrible pain above my right elbow. Chores such as ironing bring on horrible pain. At times the pain in my shoulder will flare up and be severe for a few days, then my back or foot or head takes over on the merry-go-round of pain.
Coping: Heat and ultrasound treatments.

CLOSED HEAD INJURIES
Eyes

I have double vision. Each eye sees both horizontal and vertical lines on a twenty-five-degree angle, which means that there are two images for everything I look at, one of which tilts right up into the air. These two images shimmer as my eyes struggle valiantly to merge the images. When I look at someone's face they move from three to four to two eyes, two to one nose and mouth etc. Even the tiniest movement causes the scene to split up and change. I suppose it's like having kaleidoscopes permanently on your eyes, or living life on a wildly pitching ocean liner in a rough sea. Both my fourth optic nerves are damaged. Surgery is required on both eyes. Each eye sees the same object as a different colour. If I look at the dog's bowl it's aqua with one eye, navy blue with the other; the same page of a book will be yellow-green with one eye and pink with the other. This drives me quite crazy. I am forever asking the family 'Is that thing pink or green?' Somehow not being able to believe your eyes, not knowing what the real colour is, frightens me. It must be part of my struggle to find out what reality is. Due to the complicated nature of my eye damage several operations will be necessary, and I have been told by four eye specialists that they cannot give me back my sight. They have suggested surgery. On the other hand apparently the eyes can move back to how they were after surgery. One doctor suggested that I might be even worse off after surgery.

Due to a reaction to Tilcotil for the temporal lobe epilepsy there has unfortunately been damage to both my liver and heart, and I have been advised to put off surgery for as long as possible.

Doing Up Buttons

I am not prepared to risk something else going wrong.

There's constant pain in the right eye, a kind of screwing action. Spatial difficulties are still a huge problem. I smash things, walk into walls, have difficulty judging distances. I walk in front of cars because I do not remember what they are or I misjudge time and distance. Dressing, drinking and eating require consistent concentration and I am constantly off-balance, feeling dizzy, queasy in the stomach and unsure of where I am in space.

Coping: Varies from wearing an eyepatch for reading, and films, or putting up with the double vision. In the car I wear sunglasses with the left lens smeared with clear nail polish so I get a blurred as well as distinct vision. Car travel is difficult for me because the horizon dances, cars are driving along into trees, trucks, buses and cars piggy-back copies of themselves. I often manage to block the vision of one eye by putting one finger up on my eyebrow or by holding one hand to block the vision of one eye. I'm at the awkward stage of not knowing which is the lesser of the two evils – to patch or not to patch, that is the question! I am rapidly coming to the conclusion that my best option is to wear a contact lens to make my left eye blind.

At night when I cough or sneeze I see flashes of light in my left eye. I find this most disconcerting as I feel I am going mad ... I can no longer believe what I see! I'm now using a 'seeing stick' (a walking stick). I think I will resort to a contact lens with an eyeball painted on it to make me blind in one eye. I've discussed this with my optician. He has located some people in Queensland who apparently do this, mainly for people who have a blind milky eye to hide. It appears a trip to Queensland is needed!

Sample Notes for Doctors' Visits

Ears

Noise really hurts my ears. I can't enjoy listening to music and I think I might have double hearing to some extent. Judging the direction a sound is coming from is puzzling, which makes tasks such as crossing a road more perilous. My left ear is still painful.

Coping: I always carry ear plugs to wear in one or both ears, depending on where I am.

Balance

Nausea, dizziness. I am still very unstable on my feet until I get my 'land legs', especially first thing in the morning or if I stand from a sitting position. Unfortunately just a twist of the head can set me off-balance again.

Coping: In rehab I was taught to feel buildings etc to get around. Only recently a neurophysio suggested that I try using a stick. This has been the greatest breakthrough for me. I know where I am in space with the stick in my right hand (my left is worse than useless), and have confidence to walk in this constantly topsy-turvy world. What's more, people do not treat me as if I'm drunk. For the nausea eating helps (the nausea, but not my waistline). My daughter bought me a couple of pairs of fine leather gloves. This has been wonderful because I don't damage my hands when I feel my way about, and I don't feel 'unclean' from touching fences, walls and lamp posts.

As time has progressed I have found that doing some 'nifty' dance steps with my feet helps me regain my balance. I suppose it looks a little weird.

Doing Up Buttons

Temporal lobe epilepsy
At times I feel like a headless chook. Reality and the imaginary are confused; I experience *déjà vu*, smell burning rubber, and experience vivid amazing technicolour 'trips', 'day-mares' that are more real than life. My tongue and the insides of my cheeks are painfully bitten. The nips to my tongue when I'm asleep are so sharp that I wake up.

Unfortunately I forget what I'm doing after I've had an episode. Several times a week I still have 'trips', when I check the dishwasher to see what's burnt, *déjà vu*, or forget where I'm going, what day it is or what's happening. I have great difficulty concentrating for any length of time.

Coping: I tell myself the trips only take a few seconds but I don't like the smell of burning, and am further confused with what reality is. Unfortunately after the violent reaction to epilepsy drugs I have a lot of pain in my heart. This stops me from embarking on a series of eye operations. This whole business has made me rather afraid.

Difficulty with perception
I skip back to the past: I look for door knobs and light switches where they had been ten years ago. I couldn't remember my name a few months ago, then thought my name was my maiden name. I've caught myself daydreaming about the time when I'm married – I've only been married twenty-seven years!

I have difficulty recognising normal things such as trains, cars, boom-gates, lipstick or an egg-slide when they are in front of me. I have enormous difficulty recognising things that are lower than my line of vision. This means I need to sit on

Sample Notes for Doctors' Visits

the floor in order to recognise things in cupboards.

I have great difficulty when I have to make a decision quickly about the appropriate thing to do. Often I walk under the boom-gate at the crossing, push through children coming out a door at school or knock children over in the playground if I don't see them on my left side. Another day I was waiting on the pavement for the traffic lights to turn green so I could cross the road. When the lights turned green I deliberately dropped my handbag. Unbelievable though it seems, the message my brain gave me was that the appropriate action to take when the light turns green is to drop your bag!

I see things that don't exist or misinterpret objects, for instance, car tail lights appear to be cigarette ash.

There's a lack of understanding of size or proportion. Trying to figure out the right amount of food to prepare or how many flowers to pick to put in a vase etc.

There's also a lack of understanding about what is the 'correct' way to behave. I've 'chatted up' taxi drivers, and I have an uneasy feeling that I'm saying too much, not enough, speaking too loudly, repeating myself or behaving inappropriately.

I'm intolerant, rude, I have a tendency to 'do my block' or even swear. This is particularly distressing because I do not know myself. I can't trust myself to do the right thing in a crisis. These problems make teaching a strain as I have to put a great effort in remaining calm and patient. With the double moving image and associated noise and distractions I cannot handle being in a class of twenty-eight children but I can cope, with a great deal of effort, in a class of ten.

There's the spatial difficulty – not knowing where my

Doing Up Buttons

mouth is, how to stand straight, sit in the middle of a chair and not fall off, or lie in the middle of the physio's couch, walking into door-jambs, walls etc. I cannot judge distances. I am frightened because the ground seems so far away. I constantly break things.

I am training myself to understand time again, how long it takes to do certain tasks by constantly giving myself little guessing tests and checking against my watch repeatedly. I became aware that digital time meant little to me, so I put a large-faced analogue clock in the kitchen instead of depending on the small digital clock on the stove. This has helped me 'see' time moving around the face of the clock – diagrams, pictures and movements somehow 'speak' to me more clearly than words and numbers.

I always had a compass in my head and a sure nose at finding my way around. Now I experience hopelessness even trying to find which direction to go in when I visit the hospital for classes, or in the city or a large store. To cope, I ask for directions, but this in itself is a daunting task as I can't depend on my mouth to say what I want it to say!

I am confused that there are no longer pounds, shillings and pence. I have been tricked by shopkeepers, taxi drivers: when counting out change they can give me a five-dollar note and I believe that they have given me a twenty-dollar note. I had a heart-rending experience once when buying a book from a disabled person. I was not sure if I gave him a fifty-dollar or ten-dollar note. Talk about the blind leading the blind! After counting all his takings for the day we discovered I'd given him fifty dollars, but I still couldn't work out what change I needed. This was a most mortifying experience in front of a shop full of people. I am never sure if I have been given the right change, or how much several articles will cost. Shopping is no longer easy!

Coping: With my short-term memory I constantly forget what my problems are, so I have to face the fact that I'm 'different'. I don't think that I have accepted that I am different yet, so I give myself little tests to prove that I'm OK, for example, setting the table – only to end up being bitterly disappointed when I can't remember that it's an extra knife I need.

It has been a relief to read that these experiences are 'normal' for head-injured people. This makes the process easier to bear – I am not mad or crazy or stupid; it's OK to have these weird troubles.

The very spasmodic nature of these difficulties makes the coping process so difficult. I constantly feel as if I am walking along a fence with knot holes in it: you only get brief glimpses of what is behind the fence and you have to guess at the whole by just viewing isolated, unrelated fragments.

Short and long-term memory difficulties
My short-term memory is very poor. At school I cannot remember students' names, which is sad and embarrassing as the students link remembering names with liking them. In three terms I only remembered one new name. Names of students I have taught before are generally pretty easy, with a few slips now and then.

I also cannot remember what I taught in a previous lesson or, if I am interrupted, what has gone before in the lesson. I repeat myself to family and friends. In the kitchen I can't remember what ingredient from a recipe I am looking for in the pantry between the cookery book and the shelf if I do not make an image of the ingredient in my mind. I forget if I have put certain ingredients in the soup, for instance.

I forget what I'm doing, where I'm going, what is at the end of the road we are travelling along. I have no memory of so many past experiences, including who I am, happenings with the children, my wedding and small things as what colour my bridesmaids wore. It all seems rather petty, but the process of coming up against a brick wall can be demoralising.

Coping: Writing things down helps except I forget that I forget. So often I do not remember to write things down. I have found that acting helps, otherwise the children feel really sad that I've forgotten some marvellous event from the past. I have found that I can get them talking about events and then key them into my memory again. Poring over family photos are also a help.

Communication problems

Frequently I have extreme difficulty hearing or understanding what people are saying to me. I can liken it to being in France. I could smile and nod and people thought I understood the conversation. In reality I was frantically translating the French into English, processing the information, thinking of my answer, then translating it into French. Often by the time I have my answer ready the time for the comment has passed. The difficulty of translating the keyword or trying to process what it means and getting stuck on just one word compounds the sensation of being lost and bewildered. This is totally disempowering, frustrating and demoralising, because no matter how hard you

Sample Notes for Doctors' Visits

work and strain, you get left behind and look foolish.

I have enormous difficulty asking for things in shops and have on occasions burst into tears when the words 'wholemeal bread, thanks' will not form themselves in my mind, let alone come out my lips!

I cannot follow a conversation if I do not know the topic being discussed. I cannot make sense of what is being said unless I have the subject to slot the information into or connect with. At times I say stupid made-up words or confuse words. This is embarrassing. (But I've come a long way from the days in hospital when I would lie for hours making a strange sound just to prove to myself that I was alive!)

Coping: Writing down the things I want to say helps. I keep asking my family to give me a heading, a topic before they expand on an idea. Often when people talk it is not till the *end* of the sentence that we find out what the subject is. 'What are we talking about?' helps to focus my mind on the topic, to open the drawer of the filing cabinet of my mind so I can hook into relevant words.

Reading

The need for the topic perhaps explains why I can study and read newspapers: it is an enormous strain but the big bold headings and subheadings help. I just cannot follow a story or novel because I have no thread to hang everything on. When studying there are headings and subheadings to follow.

Coping: I need to patch one eye, and at times I still have trouble following lines unless I use a ruler. I have tried writing summaries, highlighting keywords, keeping a written description of characters and what they have done etc – anything to read a novel – all to no avail. I have tried switching to short stories (something I didn't like in the past), but I can't remember enough to make the reading worthwhile. I have been very disappointed with this part of my difficulties – all this time at home when I could get 'lost' in a good book! I am experimenting with factual accounts at the moment, and telling myself to enjoy what I'm reading just at the moment – it doesn't matter if I can't remember and connect things later. Talking books are no good: if I am having trouble processing a certain word I get lost. I also have too much difficulty following the plot for the process to hold any joy. Frustrating!

Writing
When writing by hand I put in silly unrelated letters or write the wrong letter. My alphabet skills are still very wonky and to look up a name in a telephone book is some task.
Coping: Thank heavens for computers! As my left hand does not obey me properly I have enormous difficulty with capital letters. My mind will say, 'Left hand, hold down the Shift key so that I can type a capital letter', but my left hand is so slow to react that I am up to the next word before the capital letter appears. Unfortunately, I constantly forget that this happens. Thank heavens for spell-checkers and sons and daughters who help their Mum! Each line will have up to three errors because I cannot touch-type or see the keys clearly with the double vision. I usually hit the letter next to the one I need.

I cannot remember how to turn off the computer or do simple things, so I am *very* dependent on the patience of my two sons. I cannot express how frustrating it is when I am home alone, looking forward to a couple of hours' writing,

Sample Notes for Doctors' Visits

when I inadvertently press the wrong key and strange things happen. Oh, the amount of work I have lost because I can't remember what I wrote two minutes later.

My thermostat
This is slowly improving. My sense of smell and taste is returning.

Depression/frustration
I am afraid things get the better of me and I have to take myself quietly off into the garden to weep, or I will sit in a taxi with silent tears running down my cheeks. The pain is great, my sadness is great also, but greatest is my fear.

Horror of choking
Flashes of being trapped in the car and not being able to breathe overwhelm me at strange moments. I cannot bear to have a seat-belt against me. Even a jumper or frock with a round neck makes me panic. Kissing is a terrifying experience!

Exhaustion
I become exhausted easily and at times get overtired and difficult and cranky, like a child.

Left side problems
As I tend to have difficulty controlling my left side I hurt, knock and burn my left hand. My left hand still wants to clench itself into a fist, this means the palm is sometimes cut with my nails. I'm not aware of pain in this hand or rather, it takes so long time for the sensation of pain to penetrate I

Doing Up Buttons

really do some damage. This has led to some terrible burns. For example, I've put my left hand on a kettle to see if it has boiled. It had, and my hand was burnt before I was aware of the heat. Another time I could not remember if the iron was on so I ironed the ironing board for some minutes then felt it with my left hand. That was a very nasty burn. The problem of forgetting can lead to disasters.

I also have trouble controlling my left foot. I experience extreme pain in and outside of my heel. I sometimes have to crawl first thing in the morning as the pain is so great. I have very limited movement of the left foot in spite of doing exercises for the past three months. I often forget to dry my left leg as I'm not aware it belongs to my body. This can lead to awkward moments. Many's the night I've showered, then got into bed to be confronted with a very big wet thing. I've actually attempted to push the thing out of bed only to find myself on the floor. The wet thing was attached to me – it was my own left leg!

Coping: I try to flatten out my curled left hand with exercises, sit on it or squeeze it flat with my knees when sitting. I try to dry my whole body, I concentrate and say, 'One leg, two legs', but I forget to remember.

Glossary of Terms
Information from Headway

Adynamia Difficulty initiating activities. Gives the appearance of lethargy.

Aphasia/Dysphasia Difficulty understanding or expressing language as a result of damage to the brain.

Arterial Line A very thin tube (catheter) inserted into an artery to allow direct measurement of the blood pressure, the amounts of oxygen and carbon dioxide in the blood.

Ataxia Abnormal movements due to loss of coordination of the muscles.

Blood Clot or Haematoma A collection of blood where it should not be.

Brain Stem The lower extension of the brain that connects to the spinal cord. Neurological functions located in the brain stem include those necessary for survival (breathing, heart rate) and for arousal (being awake and alert).

Cerebellum The portion of the brain (located at the back) that helps coordinate movement. Damage may result in ataxia.

Cerebral Concerning the brain.

Coma State of not being responsive or able to be aroused.

Contra Coupe Bruising of the brain tissue on the side opposite where the blow was struck.

CT Scan Computerised tomography. A series of X-rays at different levels of the brain.

Diffuse Brain Injury Injury to cells in many areas of the brain rather than one specific location.

Dysarthria Difficulty speaking because of weakness and lack of coordination of the muscles of speech.

Dysphagia Difficulty swallowing.

Dysphraxia Difficulty performing voluntary movements not due to weakness but because of motor coordination problems.

Echolalia Imitation of sounds or words without comprehension. This is a normal stage of language development in infants, but is abnormal in adults.

Electroencephalogram (EEG) A test used to record any changes in electrical activity of the brain by placing electrodes on the scalp. An EEG is used in the testing of epilepsy.

Epilepsy Seizure or fit activity involving parts of or the complete body.

Focal Brain Injury Injury restricted to one region (as opposed to diffuse).

Frontal Lobes Part of the brain involved in planning, organising, problem solving, selective attention, personality and a variety of 'higher cognitive functions'.

Hard Collar Stiff plastic collar worn to support the neck.

Impulsivity A tendency to rush into something without reflecting or thinking first.

Magnetic Resonance Imaging (MRI) Enables detailed pictures of the brain to be acquired using a scanning machine. It uses a strong magnet rather than X-rays.

Occipital Lobes Region in the back of the brain that processes visual information. Damage to this lobe can cause visual deficits.

Glossary of Terms

Parietal Lobes Two lobes of the brain (left and right) located behind the frontal lobe at the top of the brain.

Perseveration The inappropriate persistence of a response in a current task which may have been appropriate for a former task. Perseverations may be verbal or motoric.

Post-trauma Amnesia (PTA) The period after being in a coma when there is confused behaviour and no continuous memory of day-to-day events.

Preprioception The sensory awareness of the position of the body parts with or without body movement.

Spasticity An involuntary increase in muscle tone (tension).

Temporal Lobes Two lobes, one on each side of the brain, located at about level with the ears. These lobes allow a person to tell one smell from another, and one sound from another. They also help in sorting new information and are believed to be responsible for short-term memory.

REHABILITATION PROFESSIONALS

Medical Rehabilitation Specialist The medical registrar involved with ongoing medical problems, and liaises with other treating doctors about the patients' injuries to help their overall rehabilitation.

Neuropsychologist Evaluates memory, intellectual, emotional and behavioural changes and assesses the person's thinking, problem-solving and memory capacities. As time progresses the patient is reassessed by the neuropsychologist to measure progress.

Occupational Therapist Assists in establishing a routine of self-care and living skills. Therapists focus on your ability to perform functional tasks, and evaluate how you use your fingers, hand-eye coordination and so on.

Physiotherapist Manages the physical injuries from fractures to soft-tissue injuries or neurological ones such as paralysis, spasticity, lack of coordination and balance difficulties.

Rehabilitation and Vocational Counselling Provide vocational assessment and counselling, and support the patient's return to a previous or new employment and/or training.

Social Work Staff Support the patient and their family in dealing with the emotional and psychological impact of their injuries. They may assist in financial matters such as liaison with Social Security, the insurance company, lawyers and help to organise accommodation.

Speech Pathologist As language problems are among the most common long-lasting problems of head-injured people the therapist evaluates the patient's listening and conversational skills and works to help the patient in listening, speaking, reading and writing.

P.P.S. The Fourteen Anniversary Approaches

Experience is not what happens to a person. It's what a person does with what happens to them.

– Aldous Huxley

Happiness is dedication to a worthy purpose.

– Helen Keller

I could never have foreseen the response my simple story would bring. Invitations to speak to people with brain injury, their families, carers, support groups and professionals have meant Ted and I have had the privilege of meeting many, extraordinary people. We have had rich and marvellous experiences with our contact with the people, worldwide, whose lives have been touched by brain injury – enough stories to fill another book.

Whenever I speak to an audience of people with brain injury, I ask for a show of hands from those who have done something they were told they would never do. It's heart warming to see the pleasure and pride on the faces as a sea of hands rises in the air. I've learnt so much from these people as with humour, and sometimes irony, they generously and honestly share discoveries they've made.

I met Martin at a Headway group in Oxford UK and we regularly exchange emails

Email to: Martin Birch
On: 2 April 2005

Dear Martin,

It was great to receive your last email – to hear of your activities at Speakability and Headway. I can just imagine you working on your bonsai trees and painting.

Easter was great. Can you imagine Ted and the six grandchildren feeding the kookaburras on the deck? (They now have proof that kookaburras prefer minced steak to Easter eggs!) My manuscript for 'Dance of the Seven Steps' is with a publisher and I've just signed with a Brazilian publisher for my book 'Chasing Ideas' to be translated into Portuguese – perhaps it will make more sense to me than the Chinese version! Last night I spoke to a group of school principals (about resilience and coping with change), next week to a group of parents, later to staff at a hospital. There's never a dull moment. Something is always happening – life is wonderful. Even though my sight hasn't improved and I hurt each day, I feel a little better than I used to so I feel like I'm growing 'younger' rather than 'older'. As my dear dad always said, 'Nil desperandum' – never give up hope.

Martin, you always finish your emails to me 'Never surrender.' We will never ever surrender or give up – will we?

Much love to you and Linda

Chris x

I've Discovered ...

I've discovered that you feel a 'lesser person' if you spill your food down your front.

I've discovered that coffee smells wonderful.

I've discovered that it doesn't matter if you can't understand all of a movie, play or book – you can just enjoy them for the moment.

I've discovered that a pat can be worth a thousand words.

I've discovered that it's difficult if you don't understand the atmosphere or tone of situations.

I've discovered that it's frustrating waiting for taxis.

I've discovered that a dog can understand human emotions.

I've discovered that touching is like seeing.

I've discovered that it's hard to try to understand what is obvious to others.

I've discovered that a sense of smell can be very useful.

I've discovered that too many problems rolled and tangled together are unsolvable.

I've discovered that you can unintentionally hurt people.

I've discovered that a 'good cry' can be good.

I've discovered that we can push so hard for what we want that we don't see or value what we have.

I've discovered that you need to let go of dammed-back feelings.

Doing Up Buttons

I've discovered it's very difficult to work out what to fight for and what to compromise on.

I've discovered that it's embarrassing to be different.

I've discovered that days can seem a month long when there is nothing to distract you.

I've discovered that curiosity can be a cure for boredom.

I've discovered that little things are important.

I've discovered that curiosity helps.

I've discovered that it is important to prioritise.

I've discovered that you need to find out what's worth striving for and what should be compromised or ignored.

I've discovered that you have to constantly strive to find a different or better way to do things.

I've discovered that we learn a lot from our mistakes

I've discovered that you have to sometimes try to find new and different ways of doing things, you can't just take things for granted.

I've discovered that taxi drivers can help you understand life.

I've discovered that information helps in many ways.

I've discovered that sympathy and understanding can halve the burden.

I've discovered it's wonderful to have someone to listen.

I've discovered that people can be kind or cruel.

I've discovered that it's awful if you can't remember people's names.

I've discovered that you can resent people who have power over you.

I've discovered that you must tackle the big problem and

I've Discovered . . .

break it into smaller bits so that you understand and tackle a manageable piece at a time.

I've discovered that when you know the whole story, it's easier to put yourself together.

I've discovered that things like a shoe horn or a shopping trolley are really useful.

I've discovered that listening to unfamiliar music doesn't make you as sad.

I've discovered that you can do up buttons.

To contact Christine Durham or learn more about her, go to www.talkaboutchange.com. Christine is compiling 'Words of Wisdom and Encouragement', helpful suggestions to/from people with brain injury and their supporters. Please go to www.doingupbuttons.com to give your advice and encouragement.